Training
and Teaching the
Mental Health
Professional
An In-Depth Approach

Jed A. Yalof, Psy.D., ABPP

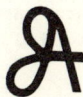

JASON ARONSON INC.
Northvale, New Jersey
London

Production Editor: Judith D. Cohen

This book was set in 11-point Garamond by TechType of Upper Saddle River, New Jersey, and printed and bound by Book-mart Press of North Bergen, New Jersey.

Library of Congress Cataloging-in-Publication Data

Yalof, Jed A.
    Training and teaching the mental health professional : an in-depth
    approach / by Jed A. Yalof.
        p.   cm.
    Includes bibliographical references and index.
    ISBN 1-56821-710-2 (alk. paper)
        1. Psychotherapy—Study and teaching—Psychological aspects.
    2. Teacher–student relationships.   3. Psychoanalysis.   I. Title.
    RC489.Y35   1996
    616.89′14′0711—dc20   94-21425

Manufactured in the United States of America. Jason Aronson Inc. offers books and cassettes. For information and catalog write to Jason Aronson Inc., 230 Livingston Street, Northvale, New Jersey 07647.

To Barb, Jen, and Brett, with love

CONTENTS

Acknowledgments   ix

Introduction   xiii

**PART I: THE PSYCHOANALYTICALLY INFORMED
         TEACHER IN CONTEXT**

1. Contributions of Psychoanalytic
   Psychology to Teaching   3

   Psychoanalytic Writings on Classroom
   Teaching: Questions and Answers   8

   The Psychoanalytic Educator-Clinician in
   Historical Context   12

   Psychoanalytic Theories and the
   Motive to Learn   17

   Learning Problems and Psychoanalytic
   Explanations   23

2. The Psychoanalytic Educator:
   An Interdisciplinary Identity   27

   The Motivation to Teach and Help Others   30

   Psychological Risks in Teaching and
   Helping Others   46

3. The Holding Environment and the
    Educational Setting   53

    PART II: CLASSROOM TEACHING AS A
    PSYCHOANALYTIC ACTIVITY

4. The Classroom Framework   75

5. Student–Teacher Dynamics and
    Intrapsychic Processes: Psychosexuality,
    Ego Functions, Object Relations,
    and Selfobject Needs   111

        Psychosexuality   115

        Ego Functions   119

        Self and Object Representations   120

        Selfobject Needs   121

6. Student–Teacher Dynamics and
    Interpersonal Processes: Transference,
    Countertransference,
    and Projective Identification   133

        The Interpersonal Dimension of
        Experience   136

        Transference   138

        Countertransference   148

        Projective Identification   160

7. Teaching Clinical Courses   169

        Projective Personality Assessment   173

        Abnormal Behavior   180

        Psychoanalytic Theory and Therapy   183

        Clinical Seminar   193

PART III: THE PSYCHODYNAMICS OF TEACHING TASKS

8. Preparation 205

    Preparation as Clinical Process 208

    Regression and Creativity in
    Classroom Preparation 211

    The Teacher's Identifications with
    Teacher Role Models 215

    The Teacher's Character Trends 216

    Students as Inner Voice 221

    Administrators as Inner Voice 224

9. Lecturing 229

    Lecturing as a Psychoanalytic Contrast 232

    Lecturing as an Empathic Intervention 236

    The Teacher's Vulnerability as Lecturer 237

    Countertransference Manifestations
    during a Lecture 240

    Lecture Content as an Interpersonal Trigger 242

10. Evaluation 251

    Dynamic Considerations in Test Taking 254

    Test Format as Psychoanalytic Analog 261

    Dynamic Considerations in
    Grading Students 271

    Student as Instructor to the Teacher 275

References 277

Credits 289

Index 291

ACKNOWLEDGMENTS

I wrote this book over a period of fifteen months while trying to maintain a fullness of family and professional life—not the easiest thing to do. What made the writing easy was the constant support and companionship of my wife, who read and playfully critiqued everything; my children, who make life easier; and my parents, who supported my educational pursuits. It was in my formative years that I began to learn life's lessons about human nature that govern both teaching and treating, including vulnerability, guidance, hope, persistence, and desire. I am appreciative here of my mother's encouraging the long-term benefits of my long-term education.

There were many other people who helped me in the writing process. I owe much gratitude to the staff at Jason Aronson, who gave me freedom to develop and refine the ideas within this book.

I also thank my friends and colleagues, Drs. Janet Etzi, Paul Sachs, Ann Salyard, Norman Schaffer, Deborah Suler, and John Suler, each of whom reviewed chapters. Special thanks to Dr. Daniel Maloney, Dean of the Graduate Division at Immaculata College, for reviewing several of the chapters and illustrations with a sensitive eye. The illustrations themselves represent a blend of fiction and reality.

I was also fortunate to have the two people who have had the strongest influence over the direction of my professional development read chapters. Dr. Marc Lubin, Dean of Faculty at the Illinois School of Professional Psychology, was a wonderful role model whose classroom teaching made psychoanalytic psychology come alive. Now, as a colleague, he continues to shape my own thoughts and feelings about the dynamics of teaching, administration, and clinical process. Sister Kathleen Mary Burns, IHM, Ed.D., former Dean of the Graduate Division at Immaculata College, provided me with a very special opportunity to grow into the roles of academician and administrator, and to develop respect for the professoriate and university life. I will also always be grateful to her for the opportunity to experience her kindness.

There were authors whose works I read at critical points in my own professional development and whose ideas about inner life were highly influential in shaping my appreciation for the nuances of interpersonal exchange. I am referring here to Roy Schafer's writings on the subtlety of Rorschach content analysis, Bruno Bettelheim's works on the importance of caretaker dynamics in fostering a sense of safety in children within an educational setting, and, most important, the extensive literature on the richness and analysis of the psychotherapy process and framework developed by Robert Langs. Each author displayed great respect for the complexity of communication and great discipline in the meticulousness, thoroughness, and relevance of analysis. A teacher can only hope to approximate this type of modeling; a student can only hope for this type of teaching.

It has also been my good fortune to work in an academic and interpersonal community that has allowed my own scholarship and clinical views to mature. Here I wish to acknowledge several individuals who have shown strong-faith in my ability to teach, administrate, and counsel at Immaculata College: Sister Marian William Hoban, President Emeritus; Sister Roseanne Bonfini, President; Sister Catarin Conjar, Vice-President for Student Affairs; and Sister Kathleen McKee, Vice-President for Academic Affairs.

My students represent an extension of this community. They have stretched me and forced me to grow. I consider myself lucky to teach them and even luckier to learn from them.

INTRODUCTION

People who have chosen to pursue graduate study in order to work as professionals in the field of mental health perceive themselves as being able to make an important difference in the lives of other people who seek their help. Clients come to psychotherapists for relief from suffering, anxiety, isolation, depression, and confusion amid patterns of dysfunctional relationship. Client histories are replete with traumas, futility, and vulnerability. Because the psychological process is subjective, elusive, and hard to track, the psychotherapist operates from a base of understanding that blends intuition, theory, ethics, and trust in the restorative nature of the human condition.

The preparation undertaken to become a mental health professional is not so poetic as the description of the therapist's philosophy. Long hours of study, supervised field work, a seemingly endless stream of examinations, research, personal sacrifices, financial cost, and the student's own psychotherapy are testimony to the commitment to education and service undertaken by graduate students in preparation for clinical work. Clearly, the decision to move toward a career as a mental health clinician and the sacrifices entailed by this commitment suggest that a desire to help, more so than chance or circumstance, lies at the base of this calling.

This is where the role of teaching comes into play. Students depend on their teachers for knowledge, support, role modeling, and the capacity to help shape the sensitive and disciplined interpersonal skills that can make a difference in a client's life. By mediating knowledge acquisition through interpersonal presentation, teachers serve an organizing function for their students. Together they grapple with the complexity of concepts, the intensity of attachments, the vicissitudes of achieving positive self-esteem, and the way in which they affect each other's lives in the present and the lives of clients in the future. With such intensity of commitment to a common mission of service, one can conclude that the mental health student and the mental health teacher deserve, need, and are indeed destined to locate each other by virtue of the desire to help that bonds them together.

For those individuals who have chosen to study at the graduate level in order to prepare themselves for a life of clinical service, there is a natural resonance with relationships and their complexities, but also a penetrating curiosity to understand and draw from them in a way that makes life meaningful. Indeed, it is this curiosity and the anticipation of what it may bring in terms of discovering more about self and others that seem to singularly justify the extensive professional preparation that marks graduate education in mental health.

It would thus appear that teachers who are attuned to the type of interpersonal inquisitiveness that underlies the experience of students are in a position to offer something uniquely sensitive in the way of understanding and teaching. This sensitivity shapes the student's professional identity and internalization of clinical constructs. Teacher and student who make educational commitments to each other strive to create a safe classroom environment in which boundaries protect the learning space and from which the refinement of diagnostic, technical, conceptual, and ethical understandings evolve.

It would seem that the classroom teacher who is psychoanalytically oriented is well equipped to instruct students from a base that embodies an appreciation of the interpersonal dynamics at the hub of classroom teaching and learning. Such sensitivity to interpersonal nuance and the role of the unconscious in shaping motivation and learning interests is in keeping with the basic tenet of the psychoanalytic model, save for one central difference: for the psychoanalytically oriented teacher, it is the classroom that serves as the consultation room. Here, the classroom is a place in which learning occurs in the context of conscious and unconscious dialogue between student and teacher. Such dialogue is mediated by, and mediates, the fullness of the educational setting in which it occurs, be it college, university, or clinic. Indeed, given the sensitivities of mental health student and psychoanalytically oriented teacher to relationship nuance, one can presume that a psychoanalytic understanding of interpersonal dynamics and the educational setting in which teacher and student function would be a perfect fit. What better way, for example, to understand the dynamics of teaching mental health students than to explore these dynamics psychoanalytically?

The purpose of this book is as follows. Part One—The Psychoanalytically Informed Teacher in Context—addresses three central areas that help us understand psychoanalytic contributions to teaching and learning. These areas include (1) the historical contributions of psychoanalytic psychology to teaching and learning as well as some questions that these contributions have raised about the fit between psychoanalytic psychology and graduate education, (2) the interdisciplinary identity of the psychoanalytic clinician who also teaches, and (3) the metaphorical implications of the educational setting as a holding environment for teacher, student, and administrator. Part Two—Classroom Teaching as a Psychoanalytic Activity—focuses on four key psychoanalytic constructs and their implications for teaching and learning. These constructs include (1) the notion of the classroom framework as an organizing construct for teacher and student; (2) intrapsychic considerations, including psychosexuality, object relations, ego functions, and selfobject needs in the relationship between teacher and student; (3) the impact of interpersonal dynamics, including transference, countertransference, and projective identification, on the quality of exchange between teacher and student; and (4) the role of the unconscious in shaping dynamic themes that emerge in specific clinical courses. Part Three—The Psychodynamics of Teaching Tasks—examines the fundamentals of three basic teaching tasks in order to enrich our understanding of their psychodynamic underpinnings. These tasks include (1) preparation, (2) lecturing, and (3) evaluation.

Through this book, I hope to make a contribution to the areas of teaching and learning by anchoring these processes in the psychoanalytic literature. As classroom teachers, clinicians, and students, there is much to be derived from examining the intensity of the student–teacher relationship from a psychoanalytic perspective. More importantly, I hope to deepen respect for the parallels between teaching, learning, and psychotherapy and for the individuals who commit themselves to these endeavors.

PART I

THE

PSYCHOANALYTICALLY

INFORMED TEACHER

IN CONTEXT

Contributions of Psychoanalytic Psychology to Teaching

As an applied discipline, psychoanalytic psychology has much to offer the educational system in the way of construct and metaphor. Sigmund Freud (1925), in his preface to Aichorn's *Wayward Youth*, described teaching, along with healing and governing, as one of the three impossible professions. Surely, as any psychoanalytically inclined teacher, student, or administrator knows, Freud was on to something.

The dynamics of teaching, learning, and administration, singularly and in consort, appear to make the educational setting a veritable hotbed for psychoanalytic application. Indeed, there was a strong, early interest in applying psychoanalytic insights to the educational setting. Included among those who pioneered psychoanalytic applications to education were Bruno Bettelheim (1950, 1955, 1974), Anna Freud (1935/1979), and Richard Jones (1960). Each of these individuals viewed the educational experience from a creative perspective and sought different ways to incorporate psychoanalytic thinking into conventional educational paradigms.

Yet, as might be suggested by the rather infrequent occurrence of contemporary publications linking psychoanalytic thinking to classroom teaching, these early pioneers appear to have spawned relatively few proselytes. To the extent that the relationship between psychoanalytic psychology and teaching may be construed as a low-level priority among psychoanalytically trained clinicians, the present state of the contemporary literature in terms of raw volume is understandable. The quality of the work that has been presented, however, has reflected a deep empathy for the needs of the teacher who experiences the classroom from a psychoanalytic perspective. Indeed, within the past decade there have been several enlightening contributions in the area of psychoanalytic psychology and education that have illuminated critical issues in teaching and learning in a way that displays great sensitivity to the dynamics of education. These contributions are exemplified by the works of Field and colleagues (1989), Gardner (1994), Langs (1992a,b) and Salzberger-Wittenberg and colleagues (1983). The highly instructive quality of these works serves only to pique the curiosity of the classroom teacher with strong psychoanalytic interests and argues for the merit of additional contributions within the domain of psychoanalytic applications to classroom teaching.

Clearly there are opportunities to advance the understanding of education from a psychoanalytic viewpoint for those so inclined to move in this direction. As it pertains to this book, it would appear that the application of psychoanalytic principles to the education of adult students enrolled, not in analytic training programs, but in traditional graduate programs that grant postbaccalaureate degrees in various and allied mental health professions is an area that has not yet been developed. Indeed, this area is seemingly uncharted terrain worthy of psychoanalytic exploration.

In particular, a review of some contemporary publications suggests a calling for psychoanalytic contributions in the area of classroom teaching of clinical students. For instance, the American Psychological Association (APA) devotes a full division to the teaching of psychology, though articles published in this division's journal are not likely be referenced in the literature on psychoanalytic theory and education. Articles on the dynamics of classroom teaching are also underrepresented in popular psychoanalytic journals. For example, two relatively recent special publications by the American Psychological Association's Division of Psychoanalysis (Lane and Meisels 1994, Meisels and Shapiro 1990), which address models for psychoanalytic education, appear to highlight pertinent topical issues in psychoanalytic training programs, but do not give much attention to the phenomenologies of teacher and student in the classroom. Although the structure and content of psychoanalytic curricula are established priorities in light of the new accessibility of psychoanalytic education to clinicians who are not medically trained, is it not important to anticipate and attend to the experience of teacher and learner within the framework of psychoanalytic educational models? The types of teacher education programs described by Salzberger-Wittenberg and colleagues (1983) and Field (1989) as well as by other authors and presented in publications that tap psychoanalytic contributions to education (Barbanel 1994, Grumet 1994, Kaley 1993, 1994, Kaye 1994), including programs that provide what Kaley (1993, p. 94) termed *"psychoanalytically informed teaching"* (italics original), would appear to have a niche in psychoanalytic curricula.

The literature in the area of classroom teaching and psychoanalytic theory falls into four broad themes: (1) psychoanalytic writings on classroom teaching: questions and answers; (2) the psychoanalytic educator-clinician in historical context; (3) psychoanalytic theories and the motive to learn; and (4) learning problems and psychoanalytic explanations.

PSYCHOANALYTIC WRITINGS ON CLASSROOM TEACHING: QUESTIONS AND ANSWERS

If psychoanalytic theory offers the kinds of metaphors that lend themselves to interdisciplinary application, why has the relationship between classroom teaching in the mental health education curriculum and psychoanalytic thinking not really taken a strong hold within the voluminous psychoanalytic literature? Theory, technique, and diagnosis understandably and necessarily take center stage in the literature, but is it not also crucial to subject the methods through which we teach these concepts, and the ways in which students experience learning, to psychoanalytic scrutiny? It is in response to this question that other questions requiring a response emerge. Four questions that explore the present status of the literature on psychoanalytic psychology and classroom teaching address the following areas: (1) the idea pool, (2) the reward system, (3) role models, and (4) supervision preemption.

The Question of the Idea Pool

Has the idea pool in the area of psychoanalytic theory in relation to classroom teaching been exhausted? Have there been any new developments within psychoanalytic psychology that warrant attention in relation to the educational setting?

The work of Field and colleagues (1989) showed how psychoanalytic theory is always moving in new directions, with new application to education waiting to happen. Usher and Edwards (1994) offered insights into traditional educational practices from the perspective of *postmodernism*, whose emphasis on textuality rather than universality appears to touch the subjective nature of unconscious processes as formative in knowledge acquisition and understanding. Shur's (1994) work on the psychodynamics of psychiatric settings provides a conceptual foundation for making psychoanalytic inferences about how the organizational dynamics of educational settings impact teachers and students. Field (1989) addressed the need for ongoing exploration of psychoanalysis and education. Rather than a diminishing pool of ideas, there actually appear to be many directions in which the relationship between psychoanalytic constructs and education can flourish.

The Question of the Reward System

One may ask whether academicians perceive psychoanalytic models as being valued within higher educational settings. Is a commitment to psychoanalytic psychology the surest way to move ahead within the traditional academic setting? Probably not—quantitative research is where the rewards are for many academicians who seek grants and tenure through traditional channels. Psychoanalytic understanding is an experiential enterprise grounded in the case study approach and is therefore not an easy fit for quantitative methodologies. Moreover, the intense interest in unconscious processes that psychoanalytic clinicians cultivate may direct them away from careers as educators and toward direct client service as a primary source of income and professional gratification. As such, the tangible reward system within traditional academic settings may not favor the psychoanalytic educator.

The Question of Role Models

Are commitments to both classroom teaching and psychoanalytic psychology incompatible? Not necessarily—psychoanalytic thinkers are scattered throughout traditional academic settings and not always within departments of psychology. However, a recent survey conducted by Wisocki and colleagues (1994) reported that the majority (55%) of program directors of APA-accredited clinical psychology programs identified cognitive-behavioral or social learning as their preferred theoretical orientation. In contrast, a much smaller percentage (23%) of program directors were identified with a psychodynamic orientation. In another study, Thompson and Appelbaum (1995) reported that approximately one-third (35%) of the respondents to a survey completed by graduate student members of the American Psychological Association's Division 39 (Psychoanalysis) indicated some dissatisfaction with the psychoanalytic component of their graduate school curricula offerings, including training experiences. A sampling of anecdotal reports suggests that some students had to pursue psychoanalytic educational interests independent of curriculum supports or were enrolled in a program that was openly discouraging of psychoanalytic paradigms.

Together, these studies appear to indicate that there are comparatively few psychoanalytically inclined teachers who can serve as role models for graduate students and comparatively few curriculum offerings to sustain the interests of the psychoanalytically inclined student. From the vantage point of present-day clinical training in graduate psychology, academia does not appear to have the requisite foundation for nurturing the development of young professionals with psychoanalytic interests. With few role models and few educational supports, students who may otherwise be drawn toward career paths as psychoanalytic educators are more apt to move in the direction of direct clinical service. As such, there is a potential loss of prospective academicians who can bring analytic skills to bear on the dynamics of teaching and learning and who can make contributions to this literature base.

The Question of Supervision Preemption

Does the relatively large literature base on psychoanalytic supervision itself constitute a somewhat veiled category that in reality marks the significant contribution that psychoanalytic clinicians have made to education (Adelson 1995, Dewald 1987, Doehrman 1976, Ekstein and Wallerstein 1958, Langs 1994, Lubin 1984–1985)? As an individualized learning experience that emphasizes the experiences of client, therapist, and supervisor as instructional content, psychoanalytic supervision may be perceived as nontraditional learning vis-à-vis the didactic and evaluative formats that characterize the traditional classroom setting. Clinical supervision is nevertheless revered, along with the therapist's own personal treatment, as a primary teaching vehicle for learning how to conduct psychoanalytic psychotherapy. Supervision offers both teacher and student a unique context in which to explore the concepts and experiences that promote skill internalization of the therapist-in-training. Because of its blend of pedagogy and phenomenology, supervision would thus appear to reflect a psychoanalytic educational experience in a very definitive way.

Most academic departments in the field of mental health have, however, been slow to incorporate didactic supervision courses into their curricula. Reasons for this delay include the status merited by the traditional apprentice model of supervision in which supervisors were presumed to learn supervision by virtue of having been supervisees themselves. As demands for training accountability increase and new regulations governing the ethical and legal responsibilities of supervisors are instituted, the need to structure a course in supervision has become more of a consideration in advanced clinical training programs. Thus, as more programs move in the direction of incorporating a formal course on supervision into their curricula, replete with the requisite trimmings of course syllabi, required readings, academic term papers, and examinations, it is conceivable that supervision may take a more definitive place as a routine part of the traditional educational experience. While psychoanalytic supervision strategies may make up only one part of such a course, its inclusion may bring additional legitimacy to psychoanalytic supervision as a bona fide educational activity.

THE PSYCHOANALYTIC EDUCATOR-CLINICIAN IN HISTORICAL CONTEXT

Much of the literature on the relationship between psychoanalytic theory and education has been characterized by an attempt to express psychoanalytic principles in a way that makes them appealing, if not applicable, to the classroom teacher. The task of making the bridge from consultation room to classroom challenges educators. Ernst Kris (1948), writing on psychoanalysis and education, noted the complexity of this relationship and stated:

> In a first approach the inclination may be to characterize it as one between a basic science and a field of application. Psychoanalytic propositions aim at indicating why human beings behave as they do under given conditions. The educator may turn to these propositions in his attempts to influence human behavior. The propositions then become part of his scientific equipment which naturally includes propositions from other "basic" sciences. In any relationship between a more general set of propositions and a field of application outside

the area of experience from which these propositions were derived a number of factors must be taken into account. The more general propositions, in this instance those of psychoanalysis, must be formulated in a way that permits their operation in a new field, here that of education. [p. 622]

Kris's remarks draw attention to the delicate but potentially powerful bridge between the disciplines of psychoanalysis and education. Much of the dialogue between psychoanalysis and education has been focused on the application of analytic principles to the education of young children. However, early attempts to apply psychoanalytic principles to childhood education were not embraced by educators.

In commenting on the climate of this tension, R. Ekstein and R. L. Motto (1963) described a tense initial relationship between psychoanalysis and education in which few attempts to deal with school children through application of analytic strategies were made prior to World War I. It is highly probable that the novelty of psychoanalytic ideas made it difficult for traditionally trained educators, not to mention physicians, to assimilate analytic thinking into their existing knowledge base without risking social and professional repercussions. Moreover, the dominance of drive theory with its emphasis on infantile sexuality and aggression no doubt contributed to whatever hesitancy existed in mainstreaming psychoanalytic models into the classroom.

In discussing further the gradual acceptance of psychoanalytic theory in traditional school settings, Ekstein and Motto (1963) noted a positive shift subsequent to the Second World War. Such attitudinal shift may have been the result of a rethinking of educational strategies in the aftermath of the Holocaust. Progressive education became characterized by a relaxed approach in which schoolchildren were encouraged to spontaneously express attitudes and behaviors. The merit of strict behavioral obedience to the teacher's mandate was questioned, and parents were increasingly held accountable for faults in the behavior of their children.

Anna Freud's (1935/1979) lectures were a landmark in drawing attention to the relationship between childhood education and psychoanalytic understanding and to the necessity for balance between strictness and empathy in the classroom. It was in her lectures to teachers that Anna Freud discussed the importance of understanding childhood development and the necessity of appreciating the need for instinct gratification in young children. Teachers who were to apply psychoanalytic principles in the educational setting were warned that the potential harshness of a learning environment insensitive to developmental considerations could contribute detrimentally to the problems of students.

As educators began to apply psychoanalytic techniques in the classroom, a few problems emerged. Ekstein and Motto (1963) cited Burlingham's (1937) assessment of three specific problems that existed with the application of psychoanalytic technique to the educational setting. These problems included indulgence of children, reliance on interpretation, and increased attention to the mother's need for analysis. Burlingham felt that these three problems were dangers that educators needed to avoid in order to promote a fruitful educational and socialization experience for children in school. Burlingham encouraged educators not to lose sight of their roles as didactic educators in their attempt to understand the individual needs of children and to prepare children for analysis, if needed.

The demands on educators during these early years were evidenced by the relationship between treatment and education. The partnership between psychoanalysis and education may have held the promise of teachers' being able to teach and treat simultaneously, but this promise had obvious drawbacks. Kris (1948) emphasized the merit of interdisciplinary collaboration rather than an uneasy unification of roles. Kris viewed the relationship between education and psychoanalysis as dealing with the process of communication between experts trained in different skills in which cross-fertilization of approaches was likely to occur. He believed that any study of the educational process must include the educator and the child's reactions within the educational setting. To this end, he encouraged educators and clinicians to work together to nurture and systematically study the child's autonomous ego functions with the use of both observation and psychological testing measures, including projective testing. He believed that both education and psychoanalysis were designed to promote the delicate id–ego–superego balance that fostered self-regulatory behaviors and social adjustment. He stressed the importance of the teacher's attitude toward students as being neither overly punitive nor excessively supportive.

Ekstein offered two papers (1964a,b) in which he attempted to further delineate the boundary between education and treatment as well as the role of the psychoanalytic educator. In his first paper (1964a), he stressed the need to clarify problems that were educational in nature versus problems that moved beyond the educator's sphere. He noted that while both education and psychoanalysis had common concerns about the need to understand people, the nature of learning, and the intense dedication to service, the work of the therapist and the educator differed. Ekstein identified the difference between teacher and therapist as one of role; the therapist's role was remedial, whereas the teacher's role was preventative. In his second paper, Ekstein (1964b) used Freud's concept of mental health as the capacity to love and to work as a basis for understanding the capacities of both teacher and student to forge a successful alliance in the classroom. He discussed how the teachers's ability to provide respect and affection helped lay a foundation for the work situation that leads to maturation of the learning motive in students.

Wool (1989) also focused on the concept of learning alliance. She viewed learning as transitional and therefore creative in nature and described the ways that the teacher contributed to the development of the learning alliance by displaying certain qualities and by providing certain regulatory functions. First, the teacher fosters a positive learning alliance by helping students regulate affect through identifying and handling the various types of transference reactions that students invariably have toward their teacher. According to Wool, "The teacher must help the pupil regulate tension optimally, stem undue regression, and temper resistance. Provided with such a helpful matrix, the struggling pupil may delay gratification, risk making mistakes, and tolerate not knowing, while actively engaging in trial-and-error exploration" (p. 753). As a second way of promoting the learning alliance, Wool stated that "mutual idealization seems an essential component of any teaching–learning situation" (p. 755). By mutual idealization, she meant that not only do teachers need to permit idealizing reactions from students, but that teachers also need to idealize their students by imbuing them with the hope and confidence needed to support the learning process. The teacher's third contribution to the learning alliance issues from the use of his or her organizing, synthesizing, and integrating skills in the classroom. These skills facilitate the student's ability to make discriminations, ascertain cause and effect, and appreciate the relationship between affect and action.

By its very nature, then, the psychoanalytic enterprise applied to education necessarily viewed the teacher not only as distributor of content, but as an active participant in shaping the way in which content was received and internalized. Within this psychoanalytic framework, the teacher's role in the educational setting was reformulated from teacher as would-be analyst to teacher as educator. Role revision notwithstanding, however, the value of analytic constructs in conceptualizing the learning process remained paramount for the psychoanalytic educator.

PSYCHOANALYTIC THEORIES AND THE MOTIVE TO LEARN

Although early attempts to wed psychoanalytic principles to education had its tension points, the use of psychoanalytic terminology as metaphor for certain learning processes had sufficient intuitive appeal to lead proponents of psychoanalysis and education to seek an interdisciplinary union and then define its boundaries. The richness of psychoanalytic metaphor as universal to relationship irrespective of context invites such bridging. As a crucial relationship that impacts the underbelly of social structure, the relationship between student and teacher makes the teaching process a natural forum for the application of analytic strategies to the understanding of the learning motive.

Exactly what motivates school learning from a psychoanalytic perspective needs multiple explanations and cannot be answered easily because of competing theoretical explanations. An understanding of how a student experiences the alliance itself will necessarily differ depending upon theoretical slant within a psychoanalytic genre.

Regardless of theoretical slant, however, psychoanalytic theories are by definition theories that unite around the notion of unconscious motivation. For example, such defining constructs as psychosexuality, paradigms of separation-individuation, and selfobject needs, which relate respectively to drive theory, object relations theory, and self psychology, each bring to the table different ways of understanding underlying motivations. Consequently, each model has different perspectives on the motivational base that defines the client–therapist relationship and, by extension, the student–teacher relationship.

Drive Theory

Psychoanalytic drive theory in contemporary psychoanalysis has come under increasing criticism for, among other reasons, its mechanistic terminology and sharply intrapsychic focus (Mitchell 1993). Although no longer the lone darling of all psychoanalytic clinicians, drive theory was nevertheless quite popular among early theorizers who searched for an understanding of school problems in the early analytic paradigms.

Using a drive theory paradigm, a psychoanalytic educator can look at the motivation to learn in school in relation to the student's perception of the teacher, with the teacher being viewed as displacement object for unconscious sexual and aggressive fantasies anchored in biological instincts that have as their original object the student's parents. The degree to which drives are unencumbered by conflict, the content of which is shaped by the ascendant erogenous zone, encourages mature drive expression through sublimation of base instinct into more socially desirable thoughts, feelings, and behaviors. Constitutional factors notwithstanding, the degree of pleasure associated with learning as well as the desire to learn is considered to be greater without ties to psychosexual conflict. Therefore, a relatively benign introject of the teacher modeled on loving parental introjects makes the learning process predominantly pleasurable.

Maturation of the learning motive from the perspective of drive theory was delineated in a paper by Lili Peller (1956), who discussed the role of the school in fostering sublimation. In distinguishing sublimation from other defensive operations, she observed that sublimation may serve defense, but is not a defense mechanism in the usual sense; while other defense mechanisms yield pleasure, they are not as securely anchored in reality, not as energizing, and not as creative as sublimation. One function of the school, according to Peller, is to provide the child with work that fosters true sublimation. In identifying factors that promote sublimation in young schoolchildren, Peller felt that the child's natural talents have channels available through school-based variables, such as exposure to a wide range of interests through peer relationships, the stability of the school environment itself, and the presence of teachers passionate about learning, on whom the child could model aspects of his or her ego-ideal.

Object Relations Theory

Object relations theory (Greenberg and Mitchell 1983, Mahler et al. 1975) evolved from drive psychology. Object relations theory emphasizes drive sublimation in promoting prosocial behavior and positive school adjustment. Unlike drive theory proper, however, object relations theory also emphasizes the role of the primary caretaker in promoting the child's ability to achieve optimal physical and psychological distance at different points in early development as way stations to mature sublimations. Whereas object relations theory emphasizes the motivating factor of securing a bond with the caretaker as defined by optimal distance and proximity at different developmental junctures, drive theory views the caretaker's primary role as a means to an end. For drive theorists, the object is valued as a recipient of drive expression. Tension reduction and the concomitant ascension of pleasurable states are the motivating forces that drive human contact. Within an object relations paradigm, the child's need for distancing, which is prompted naturally by the development of physical and psychological skills, and the caretaker's ability to identify the child's changing needs at timely points in early development allow for the gradual individuation of different ego functions. Such ego functions as reality testing, affect regulation, and fantasy expression each mature under the influence of the caretaker's support and protection. Despite concerns voiced over the ways in which the term *object* has been applied (Murray 1995), object relations theory remains a central force in analytic theorizing. Understanding school adjustment therefore necessitates an understanding of dynamics governing the relationship between primary caretaker and child.

The types of object relational conflicts that characterize the youngster at home and can also leave their stamp on adult development can find expression in the classroom situation. For example, an adult whose mother made him feel guilty in connection with autonomous intellectual displays may behave in an excessively dependent manner toward his teachers. He may seek unrealistic reassurances of success prior to examinations, despite having the intellectual ability that should preclude this kind of heightened dependency whenever an examination is on the horizon. Such a fantasy may be presumed to be associated with the primary predominant abandonment around intellectual competency in which the fantasy of being evaluated unfavorably by authority is stirred. In response, the student's examination preparation becomes an exercise in managing the reemergence of the abandoning object with such behavioral sequelae as anxious phone calls to peers in order to mollify doubts and self-medicating in order to prolong study time without sleep. In contrast, the student who has attained mature object constancy is more apt to experience learning with a greater sense of pleasure and without the disruptive fantasies that can mar the school adjustment of the less psychologically mature child or adult.

Self Psychology

Self psychology (Kohut 1971, 1977) represents a phenomenological account of the human condition within a psychoanalytic framework. This theory is concerned primarily with the capacity of the caretakers to respond in an affirming manner and to permit appropriate idealization through the child's (or adult's) merger with a strong and wise adult. In self psychology parlance, intensification of sexual and aggressive drives are secondary reactions to empathic failure by selfobjects. Selfobjects are other people whose ability to immerse themselves empathically in the child's phenomenological field helps the child regulate fluctuations in self-esteem. Selfobjects also provide the child with guidance and direction during periods of distress. Parental failures to soothe or affirm the child result in varying degrees of fragmentation of the child's sense of self. The severity, consistency, and timing of such parental lapse will greatly impact the child's experience. Thoughts, feelings, or behaviors become eroticized or aggressive in response to the reality of empathic lapse. It is important here to underscore the self psychological position that the empathic lapses are in fact real events. Caretaker empathy and soothing behavior serve cohering functions that restore the distressed self to a state of psychological equilibrium.

Performance in school may therefore be seen as motivated by a desire to maintain narcissistic equilibrium. Students whose caretakers have been appropriately empathic and soothing will be able to navigate school with much less of the fragile underbelly that characterizes the vulnerable student. Students with problems regulating self-esteem are at risk in the classroom unless their intellectual resources are such that they rarely experience any form of academic failure. For those students without such resourcefulness, a strong need for affirmation, overly zealous idealizations, and propensities toward devaluations, vulnerability, and limited resiliency are likely to mark their attitudes toward teachers (Mehlman and Glickauf-Hughes 1994). The role of the teacher in being able to provide an empathic and otherwise supportive classroom setting is particularly important for these students.

Writing about education from the viewpoint of a self psychologist, E. S. Wolf (1989) posited an intimate relationship between teacher and student when he stated, "Teacher and learner function as a unit sharing and creating not only information about the world around them but simultaneously and *necessarily* [italics in original] also share, create, and participate in each other's inner experience of themselves and of the other" (p. 378).

Cohler (1989) also addressed the role that a self psychological understanding of empathy plays in drawing a student to the curriculum. He stated:

Both as a method of observation, concerned with the study of the impact of the classroom and curriculum, and as a means for fostering the effectiveness of the teacher to teach and of the student to learn, the empathic method represents a cardinal contribution of psychoanalysis to the study of education. As a consequence of feeling understood and, as a result, feeling more integrated and more able to learn, the empathic approach is central to fostering mastery of the curriculum. [p. 51]

LEARNING PROBLEMS AND PSYCHOANALYTIC EXPLANATIONS

Behavioral and Academic Problems

Another strand of literature, one that is intimately tied to the motive to learn, emphasizes an understanding of various school problems that mar performance in the academic setting. As teachers well know, the classroom can serve as a forum for the enactment of many of the conflicts that originate in, or are exacerbated by, the events that occur in the student's home environment. Whether the student is a child, adolescent, or adult, the classroom is a setting charged with expectation, order, propriety, and abstinence. The classroom can tax students and stir anxiety about learning.

Indeed some students may come to misinterpret their intellectual competence for reasons that have little to do with actual ability. Although self psychology as represented by the work of Wolf (1989) has offered new directions in conceptualizing interpersonal problems in the classroom, much of the early literature on school problems was influenced strongly by proponents of drive theory. C. P. Oberndorf (1939), for example, recognized that the feeling of stupidity, which often accompanies subjective states of learning difficulty as well as mental health problems, may have very little to do with actual intelligence. Instead, he thought that the feeling of stupidity expressed in adulthood could be understood as symptomatic of fear of learning about sexuality that is rooted in early childhood experience.

Edward Liss (1941) also promoted an understanding of psychosexual conflicts underlying school problems from an analytic bent. Liss addressed the student with low academic achievement in relation to infantile sexuality, oedipal phenomena, and sibling rivalry. Liss believed that a preoccupation with sexual interest could procrastinate symbol formation and lead to retardation of academic progress. Liss also observed that disturbances in identification with the same-sex parent could preclude sublimation of drives into schoolwork. In these cases, a boy may come to regard intellectuality as a feminine attribute because of an intelligent mother and a father with few intellectual interests, or a girl may come to consider intellectuality as a masculine property because of an intellectual father and a mother with few intellectual interests. He claimed that for these individuals, learning and sexuality were incompatible and, as a compromise, educational strivings would have to be either repudiated or approached compulsively to the exclusion of sexual interests in order to reduce psychic conflict. Sibling conflicts, where intense rivalry or previous intimidation may be so conditioned as to preclude any libidinal satisfaction through the manipulation of symbols and ideas, were also discussed as potential obstacles to optimal learning. In similar vein, Emanuel Klein (1949) discussed how a disinclination to work in school could be linked to a variety of underlying psychosexual conflicts that included competition, anal-sadistic struggles around pleasing parents, oral conflicts around incorporation, or fear of narcissistic wound.

Special Learning Problems

It would appear that the diagnosis of school problems mandates an analysis of student dynamics in relation to the school setting. Yet much diagnostic strategy in contemporary elementary and secondary school psychology searches for the root of learning problems in neurological cause (e.g., specific learning disability or attention deficit disorder). In reality, making the correct diagnostic call for school problems in both youngsters and adults is a challenging venture often requiring skillful analysis of developmental, cognitive, and dynamic factors and going beyond the psychometrically based measures that are popular in clinical testing.

A sampling of the psychoanalytic literature that addresses special education problems would appear to confirm the value of searching for dynamic issues in all cases of learning differences. For instance, the shame-based fears of looking and being looked at may be tied to an unconscious voyeuristic conflict that interacts with neurological factors and potentiates a diagnosis of reading disability (e.g., Allen 1967). K. N. Bryant (1964) and P. Casement (1985) have also provided rich vignettes capturing the impact of unconscious conflict on reading problems. Kaye (1994), focusing on attention deficit disorder, noted that childhood depression has diagnostic markers overlapping with the attention deficit problem. These markers may go unnoticed if the clinician is not sensitive to manifestations of depression in childhood. J. M. Greer (1994) presented case study material that highlighted the ways a math disability can be tied to unconscious conflict related to sexual abuse.

The interplay between neurological impairment and psychodynamics was further described by B. Garber (1989). Garber observed that some youngsters with learning disability may present with a limited capacity for empathy, though the limited capacity for empathy may be hard to understand apart from the limitations in cognitive functions such as memory, comprehension, language skill, and abstract reasoning that contribute to the capacity for responding to others in an empathic manner. Furthermore, labeling these children as egocentric may wrongly suggest a callous character structure rather than the fragile self-states that lead these youngsters to become preoccupied with their own stability. Whereas the learning disability may receive remedial attention, however, the underlying sense of personal fragility may remain poorly integrated; the learning disability must be helped not only through supportive educational services, but therapeutically as well.

CHAPTER 2

The Psychoanalytic Educator: An Interdisciplinary Identity

The psychoanalytic clinician at a university or college is different from his or her colleagues in academe in one key way: hybrid interests have been consolidated around a professional identity that integrates psychoanalytic skills with the roles and responsibilities of an academic. On the surface, this identity would appear not to be an easy fit. The creative process of some psychoanalytic clinicians may be antagonistic to the formality of classroom teaching, academic committee involvements, and the demands for publication scholarship that help to define the work of the educator. For these individuals, professional interests and identity are likely to be centered around direct clinical service. In contrast, some skillful teachers with great sensitivity to interpersonal processes may be disinclined to pursue formal training in the subjective arena of mental health. For these individuals, professional identity and gratification are likely to issue from direct pedagogic service to students. It is in the overlapping of these two disciplines that the psychoanalytic educator crosses professional boundaries.

Because of this overlap, the psychoanalytic educator who has opted for a dual career as therapist and teacher holds a professional identity that includes serving clients and students. Personal identity itself represents a complex synthesis of—at the least—biology, personal history, opportunity, cultural context, talent, personal values, and accessibility to role models. Professional identity, as part of an overall sense of personal identity, is built on this same foundation. It, too, represents a blend of talent, motivation, history, values, culture, role models, and opportunity.

The weaving together of a professional identity that bridges two disciplines, even if these two disciplines share much in common, is different from the processes underlying a professional identity born from one content domain. In this regard, the challenges to the smooth integration of professional identity that await the psychoanalytic therapist who is also committed to classroom teaching are vast. Among the variables that help shape the professional identity of the psychoanalytic educator are (1) the motivation to teach and help others and (2) psychological risks in teaching and helping others.

THE MOTIVATION TO TEACH
AND HELP OTHERS

It is difficult to envision any successful therapist or teacher in whom the conscious motive to make a positive impact on the lives of others is not a salient factor that shapes professional direction. The hard work entailed by teaching and helping yields great personal reward. Moreover, helping people achieve higher levels of personal adjustment or find intrinsic value in the educational process represents a social contribution that transcends the immediate personal gain experienced by the clinician or teacher as part of his or her service mission within the helping professions.

There is, however, a distinction between conscious motivations to serve other people and the unconscious roots. According to Eber and Kunz (1984), for example, the desire to help others may be far from benign. In developing this point, they stated:

> Sometimes it is merely taken for granted that one chooses a career in the helping professions because of a genuine desire to be helpful. This view, although reassuring to both the individual and to the group image, at times may be self-deceiving. In fact, a desire to help others is a complexly determined wish that serves a number of motivational influences, conscious and unconscious. [p. 126]

Elaborating on the way in which conflict and regression can shape occupational choice, Eber and Kunz referenced Freud's idea that the urge to become a physician originated in sadistic pregenital strivings and sexual curiosity, Marmor's notion of infantile omnipotence, and Racker's comments about unconscious masochism. These observations would appear to warrant a close study of the variables that influence a professional identity combining the two service-oriented professions of psychoanalytic clinical work and teaching.

Guy (1987) has described family-of-origin influences that may predispose someone to pursue a career as a psychotherapist. Such influences include the need for emotional intimacy and closeness, the presence of a maternal figure who was the central figure within the family constellation and who drew the child into a confidant role, the presence of a caretaking pattern whereby the future therapist assumed a parentified role at a relatively early age, and the presence of a mentally or physically disabled family member. Goldberg (1986) also elaborated family-of-origin issues that influence a decision to become a psychotherapist. In summarizing variables that lead an individual to gravitate toward a career as a psychotherapist, Goldberg stated:

> In a word, a therapist is molded in childhood, whose early experiences have left him/her with a certain residue of impotence in the face of human suffering. As an adult with mature life experiences the therapist-to-be is better equipped to carry out the practitioner's family script than he/she was as a child. The therapist-to-be, in face of his/her frustration at fulfilling the family manifest as a healer, selects those educational and life experiences, often, largely unwittingly, that enable him/her to feel more adequate in dealing with human suffering. [p. 58]

The interpersonal dynamics within the prospective therapist's family of origin create an admix of hurt and empathy that helps to influence a temperamental base for interpersonal sensitivity. Many of the interpersonal skills that are needed in order for someone to mature into a solid psychotherapist are rooted within the family constellation. Guy (1987) has presented a category of factors that motivate an individual to become a psychotherapist. Because Guy's exemplars are descriptive rather than theoretical, they appear to lend themselves to creative application both within and outside the therapy domain. Seven of Guy's variables are (1) curiosity and inquisitiveness, (2) ability to listen, (3) empathy and understanding, (4) capacity for self-denial, (5) tolerance for ambiguity, (6) tolerance of intimacy, and (7) comfort with power.

Curiosity and Inquisitiveness

The Psychoanalytic Therapist

Therapists have great deal of curiosity about human experience. They inquire about it, critique it, and search for strategies to ameliorate suffering. As a subset of therapists, psychoanalytic practitioners would appear to be particularly sensitized to the investigative nature of the psychotherapy process. This type of sensitivity issues from alignment with a therapy model that places a premium on gaining an understanding of psychic content that is not immediately apparent. It is through creative synthesis along theoretical lines that the psychoanalytic therapist strives to illuminate underlying conflicts. For example, the notion that a client's dream about an old roommate represents a condensation of thought and feeling about many other people in the client's life, including the therapist, places a distinctively analytic slant on the understanding of psychic content. Such creativity embodies a forestalling of immediate conclusions in the service of curiosity about what lies beneath the surface.

The Psychoanalytic Teacher

Classroom teaching would therefore appear to be an ideal forum for nurturing the work of the psychotherapist. In the classroom, the teacher has access to inquisitive students whose questions can be a source of motivation for the teacher's furthering of his or her own development. Graduate students in mental health are incisive, observant, and eager to challenge the teacher on the fine points of theory and technique. In the classroom, the teacher's ability to square seemingly disparate impressions or clarify an obscure point is grounded in his or her ability to listen attentively and actively to what students have to say.

Ability to Listen

The Psychoanalytic Therapist

More than any other therapy modality, psychoanalytic therapy places a premium on the therapist's ability to listen to clients. It is easy to envision the type of early life circumstances that would provide a foundation for good listening skills. Such circumstances can include early parentification issues in which the child assumes a level of responsibility for emotional caretaking that is beyond chronological readiness for such a role. Here the child becomes prematurely attuned to the nuances of experience, listens, contains, and is sensitized to human suffering at an early age.

In many ways, this kind of early life experience is similar to the work of the analytic therapist. The analytic therapist spends much time in silent reflection and attempts to formulate the client's material into a clinical intervention that is both empathic and insightful. The depth and richness of content and process in analytic therapy provide the therapist many alternative directions from which to choose a strategy for responding to the client. As an active listener, the analytic therapist is in a position to shape the client's comments in accordance with his or her preferred theoretical position with the goal of deepening the client's understanding of self and other.

Unlike active listening, which emphasizes the processing of the implications of communications that are embedded within the client's manifest content, passive listening can serve as a defensive retreat from interpersonal contact. The therapist who listens passively takes in fragments of the client's material, but is too conflicted around the entirety of content to impart the type of disciplined formulating process that is one of the hallmarks of psychoanalytic therapy. For example, there may be prolonged and unproductive periods of therapist silence or unintegrated remarks that are discontinuous with the client's material.

Even if the therapist is actively listening, the client's experience of the silence may be adversarial. For example, the therapist who is silent may provoke the client into a diatribe that is designed to engage the therapist around the implications of what the client may perceive as the therapist's withholding of affection. In the absence of a sincere listening motive, the therapist may be unable to hear the client's underlying plea for contact. Instead, the therapist fails to respond empathically, and the interaction continues its downward spiral. If, on the other hand, the motive to listen is genuine, then the therapist is in a position to help the client understand thoughts and feelings in a way that may be entirely different from anything that the client has previously experienced.

The Psychoanalytic Teacher

The ability to listen is a requirement for good classroom teaching. Good listening skills make students feel heard. The teacher who has good listening skills is likely to be perceived by students as caring, responsive, and willing to learn from students. A teacher who listens well serves as a positive role model for mental health students. Through observation, students have an immediate experience of a teacher's patience and respectfulness as a model for useful dialogue that encourages questions in the service of understanding.

When listening goes awry, the classroom experience of students can suffer dramatically. Teachers may steamroll over student questions in the service of forging ahead with planned material, may not stop to process issues that seem to be pressing for attention, or may hesitate to listen internally to their own fleeting or forceful reactions in response to a particular classroom scenario; such teachers are circumventing learning opportunities for themselves and their students.

In contrast, the patient teacher who displays a willingness to respond to questions is rewarded with a receptive class. Students who have impressed the teacher as quiet if not shy in the classroom may begin to raise questions. The willingness of this group of previously reticent students to raise questions would appear to reflect their reduced inhibition around risk taking, which is related to the teacher's creating a safe space in the classroom. And while not all questions are equally relevant or trenchant, they nevertheless speak to a concern held by at least one student.

Furthermore, when teaching mental health students, the teacher models a style of listening that is patient, respectful, and informative. The teacher's ability to field and respond sensitively to student questions at both the manifest and latent levels has implications for conducting psychotherapy. Several students who raise questions about the teacher's willingness to extend an assignment due date because of extenuating circumstances, for example, may also be indicating that the assignment itself was too difficult. Here, the teacher is well advised to study the assignment carefully and consider both its level of difficulty relative to student readiness and his or her possible motivations for making the assignment too challenging. By reflecting first on the quality of the assignment, the teacher is in a better position to determine his or her role in triggering student anxiety rather than merely considering student anxiousness as emanating from the students with minimal or no contribution from the teacher.

Empathy and Understanding

The Psychoanalytic Therapist

The ability to remain empathic and understanding in response to the various concerns that clients present defines the mature psychotherapist. Again, it is not too difficult to envision how the early life context of the prospective therapist would lead him or her to gravitate to a line of work in which empathy and understanding are valued. Family contexts with disruptive interactional patterns are typified by lapses in empathic responding. This type of family atmosphere is marked by the limited capacity of caretakers to contain the child's distress and the imposition of caretaker distress on the child. Early life exposure to this kind of family setting may lead one toward a vocational choice in which a premium is placed on developing healthy communications through the medium of listening.

Because being empathic involves an unconscious identification with the client's internal world, the therapist may often feel confused about the origin of different thoughts and feelings that emerge in relation to the client. Indeed, the confusion that a therapist experiences may resemble the confusion felt within his or her family of origin amid the intensity of emotional exchange. Professional training provides the necessary analytic constructs for understanding the complexity of exchange that had eluded the therapist in his or her youth. The ability to work therapeutically with the empathic process requires that the therapist be skillful in making reasonably accurate discriminations between self and other experiences.

Although empathy itself is not a skill specific to therapists, the ability to use empathy in a therapeutic way requires a mature level of personal development. As such, the therapist must have extensive, formal training that includes exposure to concepts for processing the various types of therapist reactions that may ultimately unearth an empathic connection. For instance, empathy is typically conceived of as a series of critical events organized around concordant identifications between client and therapist (e.g., the client is saddened by an event, and the therapist begins to feel sad). Empathy can also emerge, however, from complementary identifications (the therapist may get angry at a client much as the client's father was depicted as

getting angry at the client). The type of internal processing
through which the therapist works in order to transform a
conflictual reaction to the client into a reaction couched in
empathy and understanding is somewhat more complex
than is understanding a concordant reaction. Tansey and
Burke (1989) have offered a detailed model for understanding myriad reactions to clients that provide the
therapist with a paradigm for nurturing empathic responses from what are experienced initially as conflictual
identifications.

The Psychoanalytic Teacher

The classroom also provides relationship opportunities
for empathy and understanding. Students who seek extensions on term papers or become upset over a teacher's
grading decision, for example, require that the teacher
listen, understand, and empathize with their particular
circumstances. The teacher may decide not to modify his
or her stance in response to student reaction, but the
empathic teacher will try to create an ambiance whereby
the student will experience the teacher as understanding.
Teacher empathy can also extend beyond direct responses
to students. Lectures and examinations shaped not only by
the type of content to which the teacher exposes students
but also by the teacher's empathic read on the type of
format that engages student interest, are but some ways in
which the teacher can display empathy in a context other
than individual dialogue with students.

Capacity for Self-Denial

The Psychoanalytic Therapist

Some youngsters who are given extended emotional caretaking responsibilities early in life or who have other early
life circumstances that parallel the early life narrative

of the therapist-to-be develop a tendency toward self-denial. Although self-denial may be thought of as being a reaction-formation against the wish to indulge, it nevertheless takes manifest expression in the form of an abstemious attitude. The psychoanalytic psychotherapist has opted for a line of work that places a premium on the therapist's ability to deny immediate emotional gratification in the service of subjecting the client's material to analytic scrutiny. The analytic therapist spends many hours listening to clients and experiences a wide array of interactional reactions in response to client material. The types of responses that a therapist can offer a client, however, are constrained by the role that containment plays in analytic therapy and by professional ethical considerations (Keith-Spiegel and Koocher 1985). Unlike other therapy models in which the therapist has latitude to confront, exhort, challenge, or direct the client, the psychoanalytic therapist operates from a model that discourages these maneuvers. Primary responses to clients include a sensitivity to the quality of the therapy environment (Langs 1982b), the technical use of silence, and interpretations. The ambiance of the treatment is designed to foster a client's controlled regression that inevitably encourages transference reactions to the therapist.

Rather than react immediately to the transference pull, psychoanalytic therapists are trained to deny the urge to act in favor of examining their own motivations. This internal exploration by the therapist may take the following forms: "Why is the client saying this?" "What does it mean that the client is saying this now?" "What might I have done to trigger such a response?" "What does it mean that the client's reaction is making me feel this way?" Ideally, it is only after these and other silent questions are raised and answered that the therapist proceeds with a response to the client. At each choice point, the temptation to respond must be sequestered until the therapist has formulated the clinical material in a way that is helpful rather than irritating.

The Psychoanalytic Teacher

For the teacher the classroom setting also fosters an attitude of self-denial. Although there is some room for indulgence with elementary-age students (e.g., holding the hand of a young student, hugging a child on a birthday), the clinician who teaches older students does not have the same latitude. Yet the graduate school classroom is replete with opportunities for rich interpersonal exchange. Teachers instruct many bright, insightful, and engaging students who have interests and talents that make them particularly appealing. The teacher who seeks affirmation from adult students by teaching in a manner that takes advantage of student vulnerabilities is at risk for ethical or legal violation as well as reprimand by college administrators.

The teacher who uses students to fill voids in an otherwise limited personal life may be struggling with containment of personal need in a way that suggests minimal capacity for self-denial. In contrast, the teacher whose personal life is in order and whose self-esteem is not tied specifically to being the recipient of positive student evaluations is free to respond to students without interference of unfulfilled personal needs. The range of reactions at play in the relationship between teacher and student suggests that the capacity for self-denial is a necessity for teachers. In the relative absence of self-denial, teachers will be unable to learn from their reactions to students.

Tolerance for Ambiguity

The Psychoanalytic Therapist

One marker of a conflictual home environment is the presence of uncertainty. The stability and predictability of the benign caretaking environment is replaced by the tension that characterizes the unsettled domestic front. For youngsters raised in this type of atmosphere, the tension of not knowing what will happen next can create much subjective distress. Will the parents argue? Will there be domestic violence? Mental cruelty? Physical cruelty? Children from these environments grow up without the experience of being able to reliably turn to caretakers; they must always wonder whether the caretakers will be too preoccupied with their own conflicts.

In drawing adaptively on such early life experiences, the therapist who affiliates within an analytic paradigm strives to integrate the capacity for tolerating ambiguity into his or her clinical work. The analytic therapist is continuously moving back and forth between developing and refining hypotheses in order to shed light on the unknown. Imposing order on a clinical database may reflect the therapist's acknowledgment of his or her limitations and may provide the client with a reality that organizes the experience for the therapy dyad.

In actuality, the state of not knowing is synchronous with analytic work. As part of their clinical training, psychoanalytic psychotherapists are given strong approbation for not being directive nor basing interpretations on a limited database. In fact, models of analytic supervision draw on a wide range of information in order to refine approximations about the degree to which the material under review reflects primarily the client's vulnerabilities apart from issues that may have been stimulated by the supervisory process itself (Doehrman 1976, Lubin 1984–1985). In analytically oriented therapy, the therapist waits patiently for the client's material to take shape through the free-associative process. Premature hypotheses about the potential meanings of client material are subject to a holding pattern until the therapist is convinced that the data warrant such inference making.

The Psychoanalytic Teacher

Classroom teaching, too, has its own special form of ambiguity, which makes it appealing to the analytic therapist whose relationship with the client is anchored in the discovery of meaning. The appeal that discovery holds for the university teacher was noted by Kolstoe (1975), who observed that the main function of academic life was to foster a sense of discovery in students. Yet the teacher never really knows for sure just what his or her students have gleaned from the instructional process. Even the grading of examinations provides the teacher with only a rough estimate of what students know. It is conceivable that some students, for example, know more than they are able to demonstrate on examination, whereas other students may display more learning on examination than they are able to apply in their clinical work.

The teacher's review of his or her own work invariably leads to some self-doubt about the best way to teach and reach students. In this sense, teachers must deal with an internal ambiguity in the quality of teaching strategy, including the interpersonal dynamics that contribute to the classroom ambiance. Moreover, the fact that students stretch the teacher's own knowledge base makes it difficult for the teacher to feel fully at ease with what he or she knows about a particular subject area. One of the functions of students is to make the teacher aware of his or her limitations. The teacher may find, for example, that a student has answered an examination question with a level of sophistication that extends the teacher's own understanding of the concept under review. The wise teacher uses examinations as a vehicle for his or her own learning, both through the creative process of developing examinations and the challenging process of grading them.

Tolerance of Intimacy

The Psychoanalytic Therapist

Because it makes the client's perceptions of the therapist the focal point of the treatment, psychoanalytic therapy would seem to hold intrinsic appeal to individuals who are motivated to become therapists out of a need for intimacy. Indeed, the relationship between client and therapist is organized around moments of intimacy. The therapist formulates the client's material on several levels, including the level that addresses the immediacy of the client–therapist interaction.

The way in which the therapist formulates material and develops interventions differs across analytic models. All such models, however, speak decisively to the importance of shaping critical interventions around the nature of the client's relationship to the therapist. Although not all therapeutic interventions necessarily address this relationship at the manifest level, the therapist listens for the underlying implications of client narratives in order to learn about client perceptions of the therapist. Many time-limited models of analytic therapy (Weisberg 1994) also emphasize the need to work with the client around his or her experience of the therapist. Thus, for the analytic therapist to work productively, he or she must be able to embrace the level of intimacy aroused in the therapy relationship and respond to it through appropriate therapeutic intervention.

The Psychoanalytic Teacher

The classroom teacher must be tolerant of, and able to work maturely with, the type of intimacy that finds expression in the educational setting. The structure and order of the classroom can do only so much to mute the intimacy of the learning experience. By its very nature, the

student–teacher relationship has a specific type of intimacy. Differences between older and younger students in
the intensity of their need for intimate psychological
contact with teachers may exist primarily in terms of
social and professional sanctioning of such need.

Abstracting from the needs of younger students, however, can provide a foundation for appreciating the needs
of the adult learner. According to Salzberger-Wittenberg
and colleagues (1983), younger students have some
common expectations about the teacher that push for
intimate psychological contact. Included among these
expectancies are that the teacher is a source of knowledge
and wisdom, a provider and comforter, and an object of
admiration. Moreover, the teacher's desire to pass on
knowledge and skills, to see students succeed, and to
foster personal development also involves engaging students in a way that encourages intimacy.

Although the teacher's relationship to older graduate
students in mental health education may differ in form and
content from the type of interaction that defines the
relationship to a much younger student, the underlying
needs of older students may be no different from the needs
of their younger cohorts. Graduate students look to faculty for direction, study their work habits, think about
ways to have closer contact with them, and struggle with
their feelings on each of these fronts. Similarly, faculty
have as one mission the success of their students. Faculty
strive to find a balance between relating to students
through the formality of the classroom setting and making
available opportunities for individualistic instructional
and mentoring experiences through such venues as supervision and research.

Faculty who are not sensitized to the intimate workings
of the learning experience and the ways in which this need
for intimate contact manifests in the educational setting
may be missing opportunities for personal and profes-

sional growth and development. Such sensitivity includes being aware of the ways the real limitations that traditional graduate education in mental health places on faculty involvements with students (e.g., large classrooms, short-term contacts with students, ethical protocol for interacting with students) can actually intensify a yearning for more contact. This sensitivity can arouse a range of reactions in the faculty member. For example, feelings of guilt can arise over not being available when a student requests additional supervisory time. The request may itself be driven more by the student's need for contact with a faculty member and less by the need for help with any particular clinical formulation. In short, the teaching situation requires the teacher's receptiveness to intimacy as manifested in the educational setting and an ability to work with such manifestation in a way that fosters a positive learning experience for students.

Comfort with Power

The Psychoanalytic Therapist

The concept of power has particular meaning for psychoanalytic psychotherapy. The therapist organizes the treatment in such a way as to promote a psychological regression, albeit a controlled one, in clients. The relaxing of typical defenses that is orchestrated through the regressive pull of the analytic treatment stimulates the emergence of primitive authority issues—among others—and sets the stage for the potential transference–countertransference struggles that touch the very soul of the client's characterological difficulties.

The therapist who is attuned to the role of power and authority in treatment will be able to assist the client in developing adaptive ways of coping with conflicts related to authority. In contrast, the therapist who is not fully

attuned to the potential influence that can be wielded
through the power aspects of his or her role and who
becomes immersed in control struggles with his or her
clients places the treatment at risk. The early-life conflicts
that may have made the prospective therapist feel powerless or fostered a power-laden parentification role lie on
the edge of expression if these conflicts are not addressed
as part of the therapist's professional training.

The Psychoanalytic Teacher

The profession of teaching affords the teacher power in
the areas of experience, knowledge, and control and thus
seems to be a natural role for individuals who are attracted
to the power embedded in teaching. The teacher is clearly
in a position to influence not only the content of learning
but also the student's career direction. In this regard,
students may identify themselves as being at the whim of
the teacher's grading decisions. Vagueness in grading criteria and other types of adumbrated classroom procedures
only serve to fuel the student's anxiety in the classroom.
The analytic therapist may be able to provide a clear
rationale for the diminished structure within the analytic
treatment, but the classroom teacher is hard pressed to
articulate teaching standards that deemphasize clarity and
organization.

PSYCHOLOGICAL RISKS IN TEACHING AND HELPING OTHERS

The motivation to help others carries with it a unique set
of risks that threaten to complicate the smooth integration
of professional identity for the psychoanalytically informed teacher. Any professional who devotes his or her
lifework to treating clients and to teaching about mental

health must cope routinely with multiple demands on multiple fronts. The same psychological variables that may have contributed to the motivation to become a therapist and a teacher can also render the professional at risk for burnout. For teachers, burnout is likely to increase with departmental leadership responsibility (Wisocki et al. 1994). The demands of teaching and clinical work place a premium on such capacities as self-denial and tolerance for ambiguity. Both the analytic therapist and the classroom teacher are, however, at risk for psychological problems precisely because of the very personal nature of their work. The isolating nature of both disciplines is a potential breeding ground for emotional distress.

The Isolating Nature of Psychoanalytic Psychotherapy

Self-Absorption

Psychoanalytic psychotherapy places a premium on the therapist's capacity to sit alone with a client for lengthy periods of time. The isolation of conducting treatment often entails extensive self-reflection in which the therapist attends to his or her own internal reactions and subjects them to ongoing scrutiny. There is also the challenge of deciphering underlying meaning, attending to transference and countertransference manifestations, and deciding on the form and content of a particular intervention. This type of internal process can become self-absorbing to the point that the therapist begins to feel immersed in a private dialogue. The intensity of such experiences in connection with therapeutic work can place great demands on the therapist and, if not monitored, can make it difficult for the therapist to distinguish between self-absorption and a disciplined self-reflective process.

Furthermore, unlike other therapy models that allow for a greater range of activity between client and therapist, the analytically oriented therapist has few sanctioned channels for tension discharge during the session. The analytic therapist may therefore be more apt than therapists of different theoretical persuasions to rely on the nurturant qualities of his or her own inner dialogue as a source of support for understanding the therapeutic relationship. If carried to an extreme, however, this inner dialogue may become the only source of such support, thereby exacerbating the likelihood of therapist burnout.

Internal Confusion

That the analytic therapist must understand the complexity of the therapeutic interaction with consistency is more easily said than done. In the best of times, the therapist works creatively with a rich clinical base and develops sensible interventions that take hold for the client. In the worst of times, the rigorous demands of analytic listening can leave the therapist in the midst of kafkaesque confusion—many data, but no clear direction.

Under these circumstances, the emotionally impassioned, erotic, boring, or aggressive themes that emerge in the context of psychoanalytically oriented treatments touch the therapist in a way that makes it difficult to work productively with the issues at hand. The therapist may feel stalled and unproductive. Clinical situations of this ilk can create a strain on the therapist's psychological resources. The therapist may begin to doubt his or her effectiveness or question allegiance to the time-consuming, open-ended, methodical process of psychoanalytic psychotherapy. There may also be periods in which the therapist feels jealous of colleagues who have apparently been able to work comfortably with other therapy approaches that help clients achieve relief from presenting problems in relatively brief periods of time (Steenbarger 1992).

This last point may appear to be paradoxical: the nature of psychoanalytic therapy itself creates the very sort of insular experience to which the therapist is drawn, but by which he or she may also be drained. Moreover, the type of clinical work in which a psychoanalytic therapist engages is usually so personal that the disclosure of how the therapist actually experiences the client may be too difficult to articulate. Thus, the treatment complications that arise in response to the challenges of working with difficult clients, or the difficulty of dealing with a personal crisis while trying to manage a caseload of clients, can easily lead to states of disquietude bordering on helplessness. Adler (1972) has described the kind of interactional process that can arouse an analytically oriented practitioner's experience of helplessness in treating difficult patients and has noted the way in which the therapist can use his or her reactions to help clients achieve new insights into their own dynamics.

Ethical Sequelae

For therapists who have difficulty reaching out to others for help during periods of stress, there exists a particular vulnerability in clinical work. This vulnerability is marked by declining professional judgment and an increased risk for ethical violation (Keith-Spiegel and Koocher 1985). Psychoanalytically informed treatments, with their emphases on the nuances of the client–therapist relationship, foster a psychological proximity that makes the therapist a very significant person in the life of his or her clients. Although the promise of such intimacy is one of the attractions of practicing psychoanalytic therapy, it must be juxtaposed to the risk of the therapist's subtly slipping into states of reduced professional competence (Overholser and Fine 1990). Rather than reaching out to other professionals for support, there may be shame connected with the identification of a personal problem, or the therapist's rationalizations may be so rigid as to mislead the therapist into believing that the situation is neither serious nor threatening to the quality of clinical work or personal life. Unless the therapist can move past these barriers, the isolating nature of analytic work will more than likely continue to extract a steep price from his or her personal and professional functioning.

The Isolating Nature of the Teaching Experience

The factors that place the psychoanalytic teacher at risk for burnout are different from the variables that lie in wait for the psychoanalytic therapist. Indeed, on a manifest level, the teaching of graduate mental health students seems anything but an isolating experience. There is room for easy exchange without the pressure of a treatment relationship; departmental members can share in the vicissitudes of the classroom through firsthand experience; and teachers need not scrutinize themselves in a manner similar to the self-analytic work done by a therapist. What, then, may trigger burnout for the psychoanalytic teacher?

The Structure of Academic Life

Bullough and colleagues (1991) suggested that the tension between the structure of the classroom and the desire to nurture can represent a potential source of conflict for the teacher, especially for the psychoanalytic teacher, who is trained to treat in addition to being skilled at teaching. Academic life, however, is structured around several events, each of which has a life of its own. These events include preparation, lecturing, developing examinations, grading, attending meetings, writing for scholarly review, and other types of professional, professorial, administrative, and institutional activities that comprise the work of a faculty member. Each such activity has its own set of internal criteria that are regulated by deadlines, institutional mission, departmental goals, and academic rigor. Structure may beget structure, but too much structure may beget a breakdown. Under these conditions, risk for teaching burnout may increase.

Symptomatic expression of being overly structured may be expressed through waning enthusiasm. Diminished enthusiasm is the teacher's nightmare. Eagerness, commitment, creativity, and a desire to learn from one's students, each of which may have been present at the starting gate, dwindle slowly in response to what is often experienced as the silent labor of the teacher's work. Activities that were once grounded in desire shift to a perfunctory mode. Intensive teaching relationships in which the teacher took an active interest in student development become cumbersome and demanding. Limited sanctioning of interpretations can leave the psychoanalytic teacher feeling a sense of loss over not being able to make the insightful interpretations that may illuminate interpersonal dynamics heightened during moments of stress with students or administrators. Common stress sources include unmet needs for affirmation by students and administrators and the absence of senior-level mentors to help the teacher sort through the complex structure of academic life.

CHAPTER 3

The Holding Environment
and
the Educational Setting

The term *holding environment* has a special place in psychoanalytic psychology. Its elegance conveys both ample protection and ample space to carve, shape, and solidify a unique personality. It is precisely the type of term that captures the essence of what psychoanalytic practitioners do—through holding and nurturance they foster an environment for self-discovery. Moreover, the concept of holding environment, because it is anchored in the mystique of the mother–child interaction, has intrinsic appeal to teachers with psychoanalytic interests, whose classroom activity is rooted symbolically in the parent–child exchange.

Is it too far-reaching, however, to generalize from the intimacy of the parent–child or even client–therapist relationship to the relationship among teacher, student, and school? Clearly, teachers are on unfamiliar terrain when thinking about psychically holding their students or being held by their school. By virtue of training, most teachers and administrators are hardly encouraged to think psychoanalytically about their relationship to students, to each other, or to their school. Yet it is exactly this diminished awareness around the metaphorical implications of the holding environment for the school system that makes it worth investigating. Winnicott's concepts of the *holding environment* and *good-enough mother* can be applied to the educational system by identifying different facets of the "good-enough" school. Winnicott's concepts are rich enough to serve as psychoanalytic metaphors for the fabric of university life that embraces teachers, administrators, and students.

THE HOLDING ENVIRONMENT

Winnicott's Contributions

The holding environment as a psychoanalytic construct is wedded to the writings of the British psychoanalyst and pediatrician D. W. Winnicott (1960, 1986). Winnicott was consistently concerned with the relationship of early childhood caretaking and later psychological denouement. Although neither isolated nor indexed with great frequency in Winnicott's writings, the term *holding environment* takes center stage in explaining both his conception of treatment and the alacrity with which psychoanalytic thinkers gravitate to the term. The phrase's appeal may lie in the humane way that Winnicott dealt with the importance of personal and environmental influences in the development of the individual.

Winnicott's (1960) paper, "The theory of the parent–infant relationship," provides a foundation for understanding his conception of optimal caretaking. In this paper, Winnicott identified three "roughly overlapping stages" (p. 43) of satisfactory parental care that were needed in order for the child to move toward independence. These stages included (1) holding, (2) mother and infant living together, and (3) father, mother, and infant all living together.

Winnicott then went on to enumerate some characteristics of infant development during the holding phase,
which he described as his primary concern. He considered
primary process, primary identification, autoerotism, and
primary narcissism as "living realities" (p. 44) during this
phase, a time when the ego moves toward integration and
can therefore experience disintegration anxiety. The result of healthy development during this phase is the
attainment of "unit status," when the infant becomes "a
person, an individual in his own right" (p. 44).

The continued reliability of maternal care and the infant's buildup of such memories are primary in leading to
this attainment. The holding stage also includes what
Winnicott called the dawning of intelligence, the fusing of
muscle eroticism with the orgiastic functioning of the
erotogenic zones, and the capacity for object relatedness
(i.e., the nascence of the not-me experience). The holding
phase includes moving from absolute dependence, with
no awareness of maternal care, to relative dependence,
with an awareness of the need for maternal care, to states
of still less dependence. According to Winnicott, the
holding environment "has as its main function the reduction to a minimum of impingements to which the infant
must react with resultant annihilation of personal being"
(p. 47). Holding protects from physiological assault, is
sensitive to the infant's physical and psychological capacities for integration of stimuli, is never the same for any
two youngsters, and is responsive to the ongoing maturational changes within the child.

Winnicott was as concerned with the mother's psychology as he was with the psychology of her child. To
this end, he stated:

It should be noted that mothers who have it in them to
provide good-enough care can be enabled to do better
by being cared for themselves in a way that acknowl-

edges the essential nature of their task. Mothers who do not have it in them to provide good-enough care cannot be made good-enough by mere instruction. [p. 49]

Winnicott's remarks appear to refer to the unconscious, intuitive feel that a mother must have for her child in order to facilitate the maturational experience along different paths. Advances in psychoanalytic theory and technique over the past thirty-five years have made it possible to reach mothers whose capacity for easy resonance has been traumatized or otherwise psychologically damaged, and Winnicott's seeming indictment of mothers who are unable to provide a fundamentally sound hold needs to be re-evaluated in light of this contemporary understanding. It is difficult, however, to take umbrage with Winnicott's basic point that those mothers who display the ability for easy and regular empathic responding are well equipped to hold and be held.

THE HOLDING ENVIRONMENT AND THE GOOD-ENOUGH SCHOOL

The singularity of the academic classroom cannot be divorced from the much larger institutional setting in which teaching in higher education occurs. From a systems perspective, the educational environment affects the spirit of the teacher, the quality of instruction, and the quality of student experience. In the best of times, the teacher feels wanted by, committed to, and enthusiastic about his or her university. The result of this positive attachment is a beneficial cycle, in which a positive feedback loop operates among administration, faculty, and students. If, on the other hand, the teacher feels jeopardized or frightened by the perception of a frail institutional hold, then positive feelings wane to the detriment of all concerned. When negative feelings encroach upon student learning, faculty and administration feel the sting. Thus, the necessity of a positive holding environment within the school is vital to the continuity and richness of intellectual, emotional, and spiritual life underscoring the integrity of classroom teaching and learning and the social value of higher education.

Intrinsically appealing to the psychoanalytically informed teacher are the apparent similarities between the good-enough mothering that presides over the facilitative caretaking environment and the positive caretaking qualities of the academic setting. Although the psychology of the mother is housed within a single psychological entity while the psychology of a school is represented symbolically and elusively through its constituents, both share several attributes that help define the people in their care. Subsumed within the holding function of both maternal figure and school are anxiety management, timely and empathic responsiveness, appropriate limit-setting procedures and consequences, the provision of physical and psychological safety in learning, and a resonant feedback loop that permits ongoing dialogue and adjustment to varying needs and available resources. Thus the holding environment within the educational domain is an appropriate topic for psychoanalytic study.

There are seven facets of an academic institution that appear to be necessary constituents of a good-enough holding environment for administrators, teachers, and students: (1) clear organizational structure, (2) informative and honest publication material, (3) safe learning climate, (4) diversity in educational experience, (5) predictability, (6) secure physical plant, and (7) positive role models.

Clear Organizational Structure

Perhaps above all other features of the educational environment, a clear organizational structure is necessary for the provision of stability within an academic institution. Issues around authority and intimacy are especially likely to emerge when people work together toward a common mission. A strong infrastructure makes educators and students feel safe and reduces the likelihood of acting out and other forms of resistance to a mature educational experience. In such an environment, refinement of meaningful educational interests, strong work ethic, and harmonious coexistence define the community life that gives higher education its mooring.

A definitive organizational structure creates roles, tasks, hierarchies, and consequences for all parties and helps to stabilize an otherwise diffuse array of players within the academic setting. Such orderliness provides an overview of how an institution works, delineates clear lines of authority, regulates the intensity of communications, and embodies mechanisms for change. Not only does organizational structure speak to individuals within specific roles, it deals with the entirety of university operations, including committees for both students and faculty.

The potential consequences for administrators, teachers, and students in the absence of such structuring are devastating. Fractious exchanges, prolonged states of not knowing, and uncertain leadership would impinge severely on the quality of academic life. What may happen, for example, if there is no identified administrator who has authority to settle debate among other administrators identified laterally on the organizational chart? What about the psychological implications for teachers and students of different divisions or schools within the university arranged vertically, rather than horizontally, on a flow chart?

Kernberg (1980) and Shur (1994) have both offered insightful and educative illustrations of leadership destabilization within the psychiatric setting and its effect on dependents (i.e., staff, patients) from a psychoanalytic point of view. In all cases, a breakdown in leadership structure has negative consequences for those under the leader's charge. Furthermore, unless there is a psychoanalytic understanding of group dynamics in which examination of countertransference is crucial to analysis of large group process, those individuals in charge will not be able to extract or utilize new self-awareness that has the potential to emerge from stressful events. Similarly, the destabilization of psychodynamics among academic leadership within educational administration can impact its dependents, especially its student-dependents, in ways that can have serious consequences for teaching and learning.

Informative and Honest Publication Material

Closely related to the necessity for clear organizational structuring is the necessity for informative and honest publication material that makes known the parameters of relationship and responsibility established within the school environment. Included here are handbooks for faculty and students, college and program catalogs, and any other material in which the university represents itself to the public.

Much in the same way that a caretaker must help the infant discover its world by setting up a reliable environment, so too must a university set up a reliable expectancy within its constituency. Although different people are sensitive to different aspects of various publication materials, all such information is critical for defining the reality of college life. For students, parameters that address such items as parking, tuition, fees, admissions, grievance, credit requirements, prerequisites, and graduation criteria are essential information that helps frame and support the student's movement through a program of study. For faculty, the delineation of such items as promotion and tenure criteria, course load, sabbaticals, grievances, benefits, and remuneration scale build a clear reality into the faculty member's relationship to his or her institution. University administrators require similar information as part of the reality of their work. In each instance, specificity helps remove any nebulous quality around the different roles and expectations that bind individuals to the school and its mission.

Safe Learning Climate

An infant's freedom to touch, smell, feel, and visualize—all mediated by a guiding caretaker—leads to the accrual of discrete memory islands that ultimately take shape as more highly organized images of self in relation to others. It is through this process of discovery that an infant's uniqueness is carved from the caretaker's hold. Such freedom permits playfulness, search, and experimentation without the anticipation of severe reprimand. Instead, the environment is perceived as predominantly safe, and self-perception is anchored in confidence. The perception of the external world as a separate entity is a time-consuming process that cannot be forced or forged through educative measures. It takes time for a child to feel trust in the presence of a reliable, well-intentioned, and pliable caretaker who is able to take cues from the child and intervene in the child's best interest. A caretaker who displays patience, permits mistakes, and offers timely intervention is in a good position to encourage the child's freedom to explore and discover itself in relation to the environment.

In the educational setting, administrators, teachers, and students need the freedom to deliberate, evaluate, and express a wide range of sentiments in relation to their work and roles. Such freedom serves the psychological function of creating a safe play space, an area with room to test out ideas, challenge positions, feel dependent, or strive toward new heights of autonomy while feeling protected from regression by the strength of the institutional hold.

Administrators, teachers, and students feel safe and secure in a thriving learning environment. There is a sense of belonging, of contributing, and of being valued that makes the learning environment prosper. Without such security, these same people may feel trapped, stifled, and unattended; they may be at risk for behavioral or intellectual regression. Because of the feedback cycle that operates within a school, regressive swings in one area may be symptomatic of instability throughout the organizational system. For example, the sudden loss of students from what had been a program with stable enrollment must be evaluated both internally from a programmatic perspective and externally in relation to any impingements on an organizational level. Unless the nature of this feedback loop is acknowledged and steps are taken to right the regressive movement, people can be segmented into disjointed factions that become disengaged.

Segmentation of conflict within an academic institution may result in exacerbation of power differentiation, scapegoating, and disequilibrium of existing order. Although such tension holds open the promise of positive systemic change, it is also ripe for a deepening of conflict. Something as seemingly innocuous as an administrator's forgetting to build one course into a schedule—an oversight that can be easily remedied—may nevertheless be reflective of a larger issue that has implications for the school as a whole. Students may react to this type of oversight by becoming angry, with some students possibly taking the liberty of making their feelings known to executive administrators. In a scenario such as this, no one feels safe. Using the omitted course as a trigger for self-analytic scrutiny can, however, lead to a deep appreciation of a large institutional issue of which one person's forgetfulness is symptomatic.

Diversity in Educational Experience

Diversity in learning implies an openness to new directions of intellectual growth, a receptiveness to difference in student need, a willingness to re-examine existing academic trends at regular intervals and to endure the necessary anxieties that accompany the intellectual and emotional strengthening of the academic institution's holding environment. In childhood, the hold of the maternal environment gives the infant room to grope and struggle as part of encouraging curiosity. In the educational setting, diversity in learning includes a willingness to introduce new programs, revise curricula, and blend disciplines in terms of both curricular content and faculty. Diversity also provides for independent learning opportunities within the context of a structured curriculum, novelty across different types of field experiences, and an openness to new ideas that alter traditional perspectives on knowledge. Faculty are encouraged to expand scholarship through development programs. Moreover, the institution's mission is open for creative dialogue and revision in response to the changing tempo of higher education. Such diversity respects the history of an institution's scholarly lineage and needs to be integrated with contemporary educational directions rather than being viewed as usurping tradition.

If the learning atmosphere is not varied, there is the possibility that a sterile atmosphere will gradually encompass the entire institutional climate. Omnisciently rigid attitudes in one sector of the educational pie can resonate throughout the entire system. Such omniscience may mask deep fears of dyscontrol, but it may not be acknowledged as such, thereby precipitating a crisis that affects a broad area of college life. For example, one can imagine a situation in which a teacher clings to information that has moved slowly into obsolescence, resulting in course content that fails to keep pace with changes in the field. Students become aware that things are different in the field, but the teacher balks at change unless it is forcefully imposed by an administrator. Under these conditions of change, the administrator feels pigeonholed, the teacher is a victim of ennui, and students feel demoralized. Academic reputations can become affected in a way that exaggerates a single incident; the entire curriculum may be perceived as having lost touch with change, the faculty member is discarded unceremoniously in course evaluations, students complain about feeling underprepared to face challenges after graduation, and the welfare of the institution becomes jeopardized. Reactive measures may then take precedence over prudent, long-term planning, in which the need to encourage faculty into new areas is anticipated and supported as a vital component of the nurturing hold within a school setting.

Predictability

A predictable caretaking environment sets up a mutuality of resonance between infant and maternal figure. This mutuality serves an organizing function in which the ability to anticipate, react, discriminate, and adjust to one another regulates patterns of communication. Such familiarity helps both infant and mother feel safe in knowing that prolonged periods of frustration, confusion, or disarray will not occur.

The academic environment stabilizes its hold by lending as much predictability as possible to the learning environment. Predictability within the learning environment is secured through a sensitivity to the needs of those individuals who depend on synchronous exchange among various leadership constituencies. Such exchange occurs on several levels and includes planning, arranging, conferring, coordinating, and accommodating. Aspects of the

academic setting that require predictability include scheduling of the academic calendar, contingencies for dealing
with cancellations, necessary time for vacation and re-
plenishment, regular hours for faculty, library, and book-
store, and an orderliness to the procession of academic
life, including admissions, graduation ceremony, and special events. Advance knowledge of this type of information breeds certainty, expectancy, and comfort.

Relative sameness of personnel represents an additional
component of predictability within the college setting.
Academic programs in which key individuals stay put
communicate stability to students, whereas high turnover
of key personnel creates anxiety in students because of the
potential undercurrent associated with the school's failure
to hold important people with symbolic caretaking functions. For example, the scenario in which a program
suffers the unexpected loss of several significant faculty
members within a brief time can signal unwieldy turbu-
lence to students who have come to rely on these teachers
as sources of strength.

Secure Physical Plant

As a home environment must be secure, so must a school
be attentive to the safety of its physical plant. Although
exposed wall sockets may place an infant at greater risk
than a poorly lighted or ventilated classroom may place a
student, the unconscious implications of the risks may be
closer than is suggested by their manifest distinctions. In
each case, there is a sense of vulnerability associated with
something being amiss. For example, breakdowns in
campus security, physical injuries to people on campus,
broken telephones, or car accidents caused by the absence
of road signs or poor lighting all exert powerful effects on
the psychology of an institution.

Any such fracture in the school structure has both

conscious and unconscious implications for the quality of institutional hold. To bolster its hold, a school needs to offer appropriate physical security that allows people to move comfortably and safely within the campus environment. Things that may be taken for granted, including well-manicured grounds, paved roads, comfortable chairs, spacious classrooms, hot water, palatable food, campus security patrol, clean buildings, working telephone and copy systems, and a well-lighted campus, all contribute to a sense of being safe. In contrast, any prolonged inattentiveness to soft spots in the physical plant can stir the types of frustrations that magnify quickly by undermining the spirit of those individuals affected by the failure to respond in timely fashion.

Positive Role Models

Positive role models in the academic setting serve a tangible and symbolic function. Their tangible function is to advise, direct, and shape an intellectual and emotional climate that is conducive to growth. Symbolically, they provide an opportunity to build on and modify existing introjective structures. For example, teachers exposed to calm and supportive administrators who govern their faculty with benign authority can draw strength from these relationships in a way that helps redefine the meaning of self as subordinate in relation to authority. Similarly, students exposed to positive teaching role models can also use these relationships as a way of testing and discovering new competencies. As role models, teachers do not perform psychotherapeutic activities per se, but conduct themselves in ways that allow the student to establish two types of potentially therapeutic relationships. One relationship operates primarily on a conscious level; the second relationship operates unconsciously.

In the first type of relationship, there is a conscious

exchange between teacher and student; here, the student observes the teacher, makes silent interpretations about the teacher's motives, perhaps does some research with the teacher, and engages the teacher in dialogue about ideas or incidents that are an important part of the student's professional development. The teacher does much of the same—observing, interpreting, and engaging the student in ways that may strengthen the student's professional identity. There is also an evaluative component to their conscious relationship in which the student periodically assesses the teacher's classroom performance and the teacher periodically assesses the student's mastery of concepts as well as readiness to advance through the training curriculum. Through this relationship, teacher and student learn about themselves and each other in ways that formal didactic instruction cannot teach.

The second type of relationship operates at less conscious levels and gives the student an opportunity to use the teacher in a way that can modify parental introjects. By identifying with a teacher, the student sees new possibilities for himself or herself, ways to be in the world not only as a professional but as a human being. Though not quite the same as a psychotherapy experience, exposure to positive teaching role models can nonetheless make a significant contribution to a student's career direction. From another angle, the teacher who observes intellectual and emotional vitality in students, who has contact with students of sturdy character, or who is subject to mature idealizations by students can use these relationships as way stations to personal growth in both teaching and nonteaching roles.

These components of the academic setting serve as the basis that helps to bring a sense of psychological and physical safety to the college environment. These aspects of the academic setting permit the type of exploration, discovery, and application of new learning in a way that enhances the educational mission. The example below illustrates the problems that can arise when lacunae exist in the school's holding environment.

A student forged a faculty adviser's signature in a note approving course waivers and directed to a new member of the clerical staff. The student approached the new staff member at a time when the adviser was on sabbatical. Given the fact that the student and the adviser met only once each year, the student assumed that the faculty member, with nearly one hundred advisees, would not recall the events of their meeting when the note was supposedly signed.

The clerical staff member, whom personnel had hired without any interviews by the administration or faculty who supervised clerical work, approved the request and entered it on the student's record. The staff member sensed that something was wrong with this process, but decided not to question the student. The staff member was uncertain about who this student's adviser was, but initialed the waiver form on behalf of the absent faculty member.

At the student's next advisement meeting, the adviser, returned from sabbatical, noted that the student had been granted several course waivers. The adviser had no recollection of having granted these waivers. The student insisted that the waivers had been granted just before the adviser left for sabbatical, suggested that the adviser had forgotten approving the request, and noted that the adviser had seemed harried before leaving.

The adviser then produced written notes of the advisement meeting in which the student claimed to have been granted the waivers. The notes clearly indicated that no such waivers had been approved. A grievance hearing was scheduled at which time the student was

subjected to disciplinary measures in accord with institutional policy.

In this example, the grievance procedure as a forum for
both student and faculty ultimately protected the faculty
member from being subject to unwarranted allegation. In
the absence of such a protective structure, the reputation
of the faculty member, the personnel division, and the
entire school itself may have suffered serious consequences.

This type of scenario, however, also illustrates the
problems that arise when aspects of the school's hold are
not adequately secured. In this situation, at least six such
limitations in hold can be identified. First, the problems
that can eventuate from a perfunctory hiring process were
evidenced by the limited screening that transpired in the
context of hiring the clerical staff member. All university
positions, including clerical jobs, merit a hiring procedure
that is detailed and regulated. Second, the presence of
confusion around advisement responsibilities during the
faculty member's sabbatical indicates the necessity of
distributing a memorandum that clarifies to all concerned
parties (i.e., students and faculty) any changes in line of
authority pertaining to student service. Third, the apparent absence of a program of study signed by the
adviser, to which the staff member would have access,
created confusion about what had or had not been waived
by the adviser before taking a sabbatical. Fourth, the
number of advisees under the direction of this faculty
member appears to be excessive. Fortunately, the faculty
member had the good sense to document all advisement
contacts. In the absence of such documentation, the student could have continued to insist that the waivers had
indeed been granted. Fifth, there was apparently no clear
direction that faculty advisers document contacts with
students. Without such record keeping practice, the
chance of either forgetting the occurrence of advisement

content or inaccurately recalling these events is increased. Sixth, the fact that a student would risk good standing by forging a faculty member's signature suggests the possibility of an oversight in the admissions procedure. Here an admissions "autopsy" would be a useful technique as a way of learning more about the particular student. Such a procedure might prove of value in determining if there had been any advance warning in admissions materials (e.g., interviews, recommendation letters) that hinted at this type of activity. In addition to focusing on a particular student, an intensive review of this type also serves the purpose of subjecting the entire admissions process to close scrutiny.

PART II

CLASSROOM TEACHING AS A PSYCHOANALYTIC ACTIVITY

CHAPTER 4

The Classroom Framework

Although developed as a distinct means of understanding and treating psychopathology, psychoanalytic psychology can be applied to the educational setting and can deepen our appreciation of the classroom environment. On the surface, the traditional classroom may seem sterile, governed by the seemingly mundane practices of lecture, note taking, discussion, and examination. Psychoanalytic scrutiny, however, reveals that these practices are anything but mundane. Teacher and student are engaged in relationships that may be structured in part by the regulations of an academic curriculum, but are fueled by the vitality of individual psychologies.

Anna Freud (1935/1979), in her book *Psycho-analysis for Teachers and Parents*, made the relationship between teaching and psychoanalysis quite clear. She described the three things that psychoanalysis does for pedagogy: (1) it offers a "criticism of existing educational methods," (2) it extends the teacher's appreciation of the "complicated relations" between teacher and educator, and (3) it can "repair injuries inflicted upon the child during the process of education" (p. 106).

Even contemporary writers without an explicit psychoanalytic bent have described the teacher's experience in a way that aligns it metaphorically with psychoanalytic treatment. For example, Ebel's (1988, p. 3) remark "that there is no one way of teaching" sounds similar to Sigmund Freud's (1913) famous analogy between psychoanalysis and chess, in which he described the endless variety of moves that take place during an analysis. Brookfield (1990) also wrote about the teacher's experience without articulating any biases toward psychoanalytic psychology and discussed the value of "teaching responsively," which he explained as the teacher's need to examine how students experience learning. He also described the teacher's needing to "make adjustments via the constant interplay between action and analysis" (p. 30), student resistances to learning, and the necessity of building trust with students in order to optimize learning opportunities in the classroom. These selected illustrations highlight how ripe the relationship between student and teacher is for psychoanalytic understanding. Such understanding can be achieved by applying the idea of the holding environment set forth in Chapter 3 to the educational setting through using the concept of the *psychoanalytic framework* in the classroom.

THE FRAME AS A TREATMENT CONSTRUCT

Rules of Psychoanalytic Treatment

Smith (1991) has presented a review of the history of thinking about the concept of the framework in psychoanalysis, with particular emphasis on the contributions of Langs (e.g., 1982b) to an understanding of the necessity of organizing all clinical material around the therapist's management of this framework. In his writings on the role and function of the frame in treatment, Langs (1982b) emphasized the client's unconscious, derivative perceptions of the therapist's functioning as such functioning is manifested through the therapist's efforts to provide a secure framework in treatment.

It was Freud (1912a,b, 1913, 1914, 1915), however, in his technique papers, who first demarcated the ideal of psychological and physical boundaries of psychoanalytic treatment as a symbolic expression of the clinician's ability to create a safe therapy environment. Within this context, Freud's recommendations to physicians on the practice of psychoanalysis included specific guidelines on what needed to be done in order to define the treatment setting and foster the patient's transference regression. Freud knew that only in a predictable atmosphere that discouraged tension discharge and immediate gratification could the client come to experience, express, and integrate the repressed childhood conflicts thwarting mature adaptation in adulthood.

Langs (1982b) articulated the underlying function of the ground rules of treatment by stating:

Individually and collectively, these ground rules of relatedness and mode of cure constitute the basis for the ideal therapeutic interaction. They create the ideal therapeutic environment or frame. The therapist's capacity to establish and maintain these basic tenets, and his or her responses when under pressure to change them, are the vital factors in this therapeutic contract. The therapist's management of the ground rules contains within it a multitude of conscious and unconscious communications and expressions regarding the preferred mode of relatedness, mode of cure, way of interacting and communicating with the patient, and dynamics and genetics. The therapist's capacity to deal with and adapt to inner tensions, conflicts, and Neurosis is also reflected in these framework management efforts. [p. 308]

The ground rules for conducting psychoanalytic treatment are abstracted from Freud's (1912b, 1913, 1915)
recommendations on the technique of psychoanalysis and
include:

1. no note taking (save for taking notes on client
   dreams and single incidents of special note) nor use
   of special aids;
2. maintenance of evenly hovering attention;
3. no written reports on patients who are in treatment;
4. analyst's dispassionate, neutral, and primarily interpretive approach to the patient's associations;
5. total confidentiality;
6. no educative measures;
7. an initial diagnostic period of a few weeks;
8. analyst's need for periodic treatment or supervision;
9. a leased hour;
10. patient's payment for missed sessions;
11. careful scrutiny of referral circumstances;
12. same day and time for treatment;
13. no set length of treatment;
14. no free treatment;
15. patient's use of the couch;
16. fundamental rule of free association; and
17. no acting out with the patient; analyst's mastery of
    the pleasure principle.

Although Freud has been historically categorized as an
intrapsychic theorist who saw fantasy and distortion at the
root of transference and psychopathology, his emphasis
on the therapist's boundary management as a curative,
interpersonal factor offered what appears to be a powerfully analogous bridge to the role that parental boundary
failure plays in the emergence of psychopathology. There

has been much writing about Freud's own difficulty in adhering to the very ground rules he espoused in his technique papers (Langs 1982a, Troise 1993), but the boundaries themselves remain a central focus when organizing and formulating psychoanalytic material.

THE FRAMEWORK IN THE NONTRADITIONAL CLASSROOM ENVIRONMENT

The classroom setting can also be understood as a series of unfolding exchanges between teacher and student that are shaped by the boundaries defining the physical and psychological space of their work together. Although differences in role and responsibility preclude exacting comparisons between teaching and analytic therapy, the classroom situation, being an interpersonal one, is still organized by a set of rules, or boundaries, that govern appropriate exchanges between teacher and student and promote a sense of safety in the learning environment. Because of this similarity, it is indeed possible to define ground rules for the teaching situation.

In this regard, Langs (1992a,b) has creatively brought the importance of the teacher's boundary management into the classroom by focusing on the teaching of self-processing skills. In the self-processing class, a student is assigned the task of presenting some form of clinical material (e.g., a dream, a narrative), which the teacher listens to and seeks to interpret around a break in the teaching framework. Lunardi (1993) has also examined the impact of the framework in understanding the meaning of role play as a contrived teaching modality. In further addressing the issue of non-transference in teaching, Langs (1992b) has outlined a set of ground rules that define the teaching space in the aforementioned classroom settings. These ground rules consist of the following concepts:

1. fixed time and setting, single teacher, set office hours;
2. total privacy (no observers or intruders);
3. measure of confidentiality;
4. ground rules for attendance, participation, grades, tests and reports, and class advancement;
5. defined fee for teacher, paid by the school;
6. clear set of topics;
7. defined role requirements for teacher and student;
8. student–teacher contact restricted to the work of the class;
9. teacher maintains relative anonymity and responds neutrally to students;
10. teacher is suitably compensated; and
11. no physical contact among all concerned.

The clinical material that Langs presents in order to elucidate some key points is taken from nontraditional classroom experiences (self-processing class, dream analysis). Although this type of class setting may have little in common with the traditional ambiance of the structured classroom setting, Langs's investigations of the framework in the nontraditional classroom have provided a forum to illustrate the sensitivity of students to the teacher's management of his or her boundaries within an instructional atmosphere. As such, they permit speculation about the role of the framework in the traditional classroom.

THE FRAMEWORK IN THE TRADITIONAL CLASSROOM ENVIRONMENT

The traditional classroom environment differs from the type of classroom setting described by Langs (1992a,b) in several ways. The traditional classroom includes such variables as the teacher's didactic lecture, note taking, formal presentations by students, student participation that does not mandate the presentation of dream or other narrative material, and the teacher's essentially noninterpretive interactions with students. In this structured classroom, there are typically few opportunities for extended narrative communications by students. For example, unlike the self-processing class described by Langs, a traditional classroom environment is unlikely to encourage a student to spontaneously share highly charged dream material as part of classroom dialogue. Thereby the teacher's ability to access unconscious perceptions of his or her management of the teaching frame is minimized.

There are some other pragmatic issues in the traditional classroom that make it extremely difficult for a teacher to monitor the state of the frame. Reasons for this difficulty include the frequent absence of any direct reference to a frame break that can draw the teacher's attention to an overlooked but impactful classroom incident about a frame issue. In the absence of a clearly stated reference of this type, the teacher must rely solely on his or her conscious assessment of the state of the classroom frame. However, conscious assessments of the quality of one's own class can often serve to defend against the conflictual implications of underlying tensions related to teachers' and students' unconscious perceptions of the classroom environment. In addition, the necessary emphasis on secondary process thinking in the academic setting, which constrains the frequency and depth of the narrative dialogue needed in order to understand the unconscious implications of a frame management issue, can make it very hard for the teacher to select disguised references to frame breaks from student comments in the classroom.

Even with these limitations, however, there are still critical moments and incidents that can alert the teacher to boundary issues related to the quality of hold in the traditional classroom environment. The importance of the teacher's sensitivity to framework issues suggests that many of the ideas about the classroom framework proffered by Langs are applicable, with minimal modification to the traditional classroom environment. With Langs's ideas as a foundation, ground rules for the traditional classroom can include the following markers:

1. *Fixed time boundaries.* Starting and stopping classes on time, and a fixed day, room, and duration that remain stable for the entirety of the course
2. *Clear course syllabi.* Developing a definitive course syllabus that allows for an orderly presentation of course material, including examination dates, weighting of exams, consequences for late work, attendance requirements, and office hours, all of which remain relatively stable
3. *Teacher's limited personal disclosures.* Keeping the teacher's self-disclosures to a minimum in the service of not overstimulating students and creating a tacit incumbency upon students that they, too, must reveal personal content in order to curry the teacher's favor
4. *No mandatory student disclosures about traumatic personal events for graded work.* Requiring no graded work that mandates disclosure of traumatic historical events as a grading criterion (Encouraging a student to process an isolated countertransference reaction in the context of a case presentation seminar does not fall into this category, whereas mandating disclosure of early life trauma as part of a clinical paper would fall into this category)
5. *Useful feedback on graded work.* Treating feedback as clinical interventions that serve to modify the student's knowledge base by making every

effort to present comments in a way that is concise, nonjudgmental, and responsive to student inquiry

6. *Timely return of all graded work*. Returning work to students in a timely manner so that students are apprised at regular intervals of rank and assessment of performance

7. *A comfortable physical setting*. Ensuring that the physical setting of the classroom is properly ventilated and lighted, with enough desks and chairs for all participants

8. *Appropriate limitations on student–teacher contact*. Limiting contact with students to the parameters of classroom time, office hours, university- or college-sponsored social functions, or professional activities off campus related to the student's professional development (meetings or conferences)

9. *Respectful dialogue*. Responding to students in a manner that is respectful, open-minded, and facilitative to learning

10. *Appropriate fee structure*. Setting course tuition and teacher remuneration fairly and in keeping with local community standards for similar curricular activities

11. *Relative confidentiality*. Not discussing a student's problems, should a teacher be aware of any, in front of the class, outside the limits imposed by formal, school-based publications (catalog, handbook), or in a manner not in keeping with the evaluative nature of teaching faculty and departmental review of student progress (Submitting grades to the academic registrar and academic-departmental reviewing of student progress are two examples of situations in which the teacher may communicate personal or academic concerns about a student that may fall into the category of relative confidentiality within the operating param-

eters of a college or university training program. Relative confidentiality also means that classes are neither audio recorded nor video recorded save for special circumstances [a student requests and receives special permission to record a class])

12. *Formal course evaluation by students*. Providing students with an opportunity to anonymously evaluate the quality of instruction and other merits of the course

The teacher's sensitivity to these ground rules and genuine efforts to keep the frame reasonably stable can help to promote a well-defined and positive image of the teacher to students. Positive, introjective identifications with teachers who are sensitive to the various dimensions of boundary that structure the classroom experience help to create a safe learning environment for students. In contrast, an insensitivity to the ground rules of teaching can hinder the learning experience.

Fixed Time Boundaries

The teacher's sensitivity to time boundaries in the classroom is important because students pay course tuition with the explicit assumption that they will receive a stipulated period of time with the teacher. The teacher has the specific responsibility to be present to students for this time frame. In cases when the teacher is significantly late to a class, ends a class unusually early, or keeps a class unnecessarily late, students may have conscious and unconscious perceptions of the teacher that show uncanny sensitivity to the teacher's ability to manage time boundaries. Moreover, teacher and student may be reactive to even subtle modifications in time boundaries in a way that affects the classroom experience.

A teacher arrived only a few minutes late for class. Soon after beginning to lecture from prepared notes, the teacher digressed and offered a therapy vignette that focused on clinical issues in dealing with client lateness to a session. At the time of the digression, the teacher had no conscious awareness of the relationship between having started class late and the selection of this particular vignette to share with the class.

During a brief intermission, however, the teacher reflected on the first part of class and became aware of the connection between starting class late (the teacher was aware of starting late, but no student in the class had mentioned the lateness during the first part of the class) and the presentation of the vignette about the client's lateness. The teacher began the second half of class by mentioning the relationship between these two incidents, noting how the presentation of clinical management of client lateness unconsciously defended against the teacher's own guilt about being late to class.

Following the teacher's comments, a few students revealed that they had indeed been aware of the teacher's lateness. The teacher was able to draw on this incident and integrate it with lecture material. The next class began on time with a student selecting a problematic example from class readings that were assigned for this class period. The example that was chosen seemed to be related thematically to the teacher's lateness in arriving at the previous class (it involved acting out). The spontaneous selection of this example seemed to reflect a dynamic process in which the implications of the teacher's lateness continued to resonate on a deep level for at least one student, and probably for other students as well.

This example appears to highlight four issues related to the classroom framework and the management of time boundaries by the teacher. First, it displays the sensitivity of students to the teacher's management of time boundaries in the classroom. From this vignette, it is clear that students were quite observant of the time of the teacher's arrival not only because they wished to get their money's worth from a course, but because lateness spoke on a deeper level to an unconscious perception of the teacher's functioning. Second, the example illustrates the awkwardness that students feel about directly representing aspects of the teacher's behavior that seem somewhat dysfunctional. In this case, students were indeed aware of, if not annoyed by, the teacher's lateness, but were hesitant to mention this fact at the start of the class. It was only after the teacher had introduced lateness into the classroom presentation that students were able to comment that they had been attuned to the teacher's lateness at the beginning of the class period. Third, the example also reveals the relief that students feel when the teacher is able to identify and work with his or her own frame management issues creatively and in a way that informs the lecture process. The teacher's openness gave students room to voice their reactions to the lateness in a way that permitted necessary and appropriate discharge of tension in relation to the teacher's management of the time boundary. Fourth, the student's selection of an example from the assigned readings that appeared to unconsciously ascribe an acting-out quality to the teacher's lateness suggests that student dynamics within a classroom may be understood as including an ongoing processing of deeper implications of the teacher's frame management. The fact that the teacher was able to identify and talk about the implications of the lateness vis-à-vis the instructional vignette that had been presented to the class gave students the room to continue to work over, through metaphor, the deep implications of the lateness.

Clear Course Syllabi

Much like the therapist's delineation of the ground rules of treatment in the first session, the teacher provides the class with a syllabus that outlines the parameters of the course. The course syllabus is the teacher's statement to students about the nature and direction of the course. Ideally, the syllabus contains sufficient information about the course to anticipate and answer many of the questions that students have about structure, objectives, expectations, and grading. A syllabus that is organized, specific, and detailed represents a clear communication from the teacher that speaks to the needs of students. Davis (1993) has provided very useful guidelines for constructing a thorough course syllabus. An unclear syllabus presents an ambiguous message to students that can have ramifications for the teacher's work.

A teacher gave students a take-home assignment with the implicit understanding that students would work alone. When it appeared that a few students had worked together, the teacher was faced with a dilemma about how to interpret student grades. The fact that they had worked together was interpreted by the teacher as an indicator that there was some confusion about the meaning of the task.

The teacher decided to approach a few members of the class in order to better assess the situation and was informed that some students had made a distinction between *assignment* as a collaborative learning opportunity and *examination* as a noncollaborative activity. A series of discussions then ensued around what was and was not made clear on the course syllabus. Because this distinction was not spelled out on the syllabus, the teacher felt obliged to ultimately honor the interpretation ascribed by students to this learning task. Subsequent course syllabi clearly identified all graded work as *examination* in order to shore up this particular aspect of the course framework.

This example illustrates the potential problems caused by a teacher's vagueness in task direction. The teacher's willingness to learn from student feedback and criticism can bring new clarity to the course syllabus and reduce the chance that the teacher's intent will be misinterpreted.

Teacher's Limited Personal Disclosures

The pros and cons of self-disclosing to therapy clients have been a source of debate in the analytic literature (Tansey and Burke 1989) since Freud's writings on analytic technique. Freud (1912b) discussed the importance of refraining from self-disclosure in order to safeguard the transference by fostering projections onto the therapist in the relative absence of any reality cues. The implicit assumption for limiting self-disclosure is the risk of overstimulating the patient and taking up the patient's therapy space with personal revelations that reflect the therapist's underlying anxieties about specific clinical material. Smith (1991) has illustrated the potentially detrimental consequences to a patient when the therapist is unable to maintain relative neutrality while conducting the treatment.

In the classroom, the teacher's judicious use of selected clinical and training experiences that helped shape his or her professional development and that are integrated with didactic material can demystify the teacher to students and strengthen their identification with the teacher as practitioner. Students often state on evaluations that the teacher's willingness to share some of his or her clinical experiences was very helpful in making lecture material lively.

The disguised disclosure of case fragments in order to exemplify specific clinical issues in relation to lecture content is qualitatively different from the teacher's spontaneous revelations about the nuances of his or her private life. Personal disclosures about the teacher's problems or about the dynamics of significant others in the teacher's life can make students feel uncomfortable, overstimulated, and uncertain about how to respond. It is worthwhile for the teacher to refrain from disclosures of a personal nature despite feeling pressure to share such information with students.

A student requested an appointment with a teacher as a get-to-know-you meeting. The student had taken classes with the teacher but felt that the teacher was still a mystery on a personal level. The teacher was under the impression that the student wanted to know more about the teacher's professional training and experiences and that this request was related to the student's own professional development and the course material. The teacher therefore defined the meeting as embodying elements of advisement, mentoring, and tutoring.

Soon after the meeting began, the student started asking what the teacher felt were personal questions. While seemingly innocuous, they addressed aspects of the teacher's private life that had no immediate relevance to the teacher's work with the student. The teacher respectfully declined to answer and gave the student an appropriate rationale that the student understood and appreciated. Conversation then shifted to the student's own aspirations. In the context of responding, the student made reference to a positive role model whose integrity had strongly influenced the student's current career direction.

In this example, the teacher was able to refrain from disclosing personal content that had no immediate bearing on the student's professional development. For example, knowing the names of the teacher's children or the teacher's age were pieces of information that the teacher did not perceive as being relevant to the relationship with this student at this point in time. The student's subsequent remark about a previous teacher who had been a model of integrity suggested, indirectly, that the present teacher had demonstrated a measure of integrity by declining to respond to the personal questions.

No Mandatory Student Disclosures about Traumatic Personal Events for Graded Work

Almost all courses taken by students during their professional training are required courses. The course catalog describes required and elective courses in a way that provides students with sufficient information about the curriculum so that they can make an informed decision about whether a specific curriculum meets their needs. In the absence of any statements requiring self-disclosure as part of grading criteria in courses, students may feel vulnerable when informed subsequent to program entry that a particular course mandates self-disclosure.

In mental health training programs, there is the likelihood that students on field sites will divulge some personal information to site supervisors and to peers in a seminar as a way of receiving assistance and support with case work. Aside from this exception, however, the imposition of self-disclosure can unsettle students. Ideally, if a teacher offers an assignment that requires self-disclosure, an alternate assignment is offered to students who are disinclined to reveal intimate aspects of their personal history to a teacher with whom they have no established relationship grounded in trust. The offering of an alternative assignment demonstrates the teacher's flexibility and empathy in response to student anxiety.

A group of students took a course in which disclosures about significant others was one part of a graded assignment. Following the first class session, several students balked openly at the requirement, stating that they were uneasy about making such revelations. In response to student concern, the teacher constructed an alternate assignment that gave students the option of creating fictitious data in order to complete the work. The students were as a whole appreciative of this option and were able to use it in a way that permitted integration of important course material without experiencing unnecessary stress associated with the requirement of self-disclosure. Student course evaluations highlighted this point.

This example provides support for the notion that the requirement of forced disclosure in a didactic course can be disturbing to students and that creative alternatives born from student–teacher collaboration can reduce student anxieties and enhance motivation to complete assignments. This example appears to further suggest that the opportunity for students to voice anxiety about self-disclosing is expanded when the teacher's response is timely and without adverse consequence.

Useful Feedback on Graded Work

One of the most stressful moments for students is the anticipation of receiving feedback from the teacher. Such feedback may take the form of getting tests back, receiving papers back with comments, getting verbal and written reviews of either simulated role play or clinical work with real clients, or waiting nervously for final grades to arrive in the mail. All graded work and any teacher commentary accompanying this work represent a communication to students about their presumed level of mastery over important concepts in an area central to their professional development.

In this regard, feedback to students shares a common bond with analytic interpretation in that both seek to foster integration of experience through timely and appropriate intervention. Another aspect of this commonality involves the conscious and unconscious meanings attached to this feedback. Students, for example, may feel strengthened, wounded, angered, or confused by the quality of teacher feedback scrawled on the margins of a term paper or examination. Such feedback may be interpreted as reflecting teacher favoritism (as when students compare teacher feedback with each other) or apathy (as when the teacher responds with a letter grade but very few qualitative remarks after reading a term paper over which the student has fretted for weeks).

Apparent here are the similarities between student reactions to teacher feedback and the different meanings that therapy clients ascribe to analytic interventions. Optimally, the teacher's feedback to students is presented in a way that is supportive of work effort, neutral in tone, and balanced in critique so that strengths are acknowledged and areas in need of further development are identified. Like the analytic situation in which client and therapist discover meaning through analysis of different layers of dialogue, there are two realities that forge the meaning of feedback to students. First there is the manifest content of the teacher's feedback. This feedback may be supportive, discouraging, admonishing, vague, uninformative, or some combination thereof. The second reality embraces the student's unique sensitivities. That is, what does it mean for this student to receive this feedback from this teacher at this point in time? It is here that the interpretation imposed by the student on the teacher's feedback colors conscious and unconscious meanings of academic performance. Brookfield (1990) addressed the importance of being aware of student histories and backgrounds in order to promote self-confidence in the classroom. Situations in which a teacher may be expected to have familiarity with the unique circumstances that render a particular student vulnerable to specific types of instructional critique are difficult to identify. Indeed, save for those situations in which the student discloses information directly to the teacher or the teacher becomes aware of a student's sensitivities in the context of departmental deliberation, the teacher has no real way of knowing just how a certain comment about the quality of a student's work may resonate for that student. The process through which such familiarity is achieved can, however, be very instructive in directing the nature of future feedback and critique of the student's work.

A student handed in a paper which the teacher critiqued in detail. The overall quality of the paper was excellent, a point that the teacher noted, and the critique focused primarily on alternative ways of articulating key points. In an attempt to provide examples of how to revise central ideas, the teacher rewrote a few of the student's paragraphs.

The teacher returned the papers to class, but noticed that this student was late to leave the classroom. The student then approached the teacher and asked to talk about the paper. Because this student tended to be quiet in class, the teacher was surprised at the request to talk about the assignment. The student was pleased with the teacher's having praised the quality of the paper, but did not expect that the teacher would take the time to offer detailed revisions of key ideas amid a volume of papers to grade. The student then expressed appreciation for

the teacher's willingness to offer input and especially
for the supportive tone in which the comments had
been couched. The student went on to talk about how
written assignments create high levels of anxiety and
shared some personal information that helped the
teacher develop a deeper understanding of why the
student was both surprised to receive, and appreciative
of, a critique that was sensitive, instructive, and useful.

This example helps to highlight the clinical implications
of presenting feedback to students and the delicate nature
of this process. It also depicts how mastery strivings tied
to the student's own personal history are engaged by class
assignments and teacher feedback. Indeed, teacher acknowledgment of student work effort can provide the
needed psychic supports for students to integrate other
evaluative comments from the teacher.

Timely Return of All Graded Work

The importance of returning work to students on time can
be understood as being metaphorically akin to the importance of timely responsiveness on the part of the primary
caregiver. Students anxiously await feedback on their
performance on a test or an examination. Ideally, the
teacher is able to give students a date by which papers or
examinations will be graded so that students know when
to expect feedback. This type of planning appears to be
especially relevant in classes where a final examination is
cumulative in nature. Students taking a cumulative final
examination need to receive feedback on formative measures in a timely manner in order to integrate feedback in
preparation for the final examination.

Teachers who return work within a reasonable time
period foster a sense of predictability and take a step in the
direction of helping students feel secure in the course. If

the timing of this feedback is prolonged, it may impair optimal learning states. Students who anticipate getting a test back on a certain date only to find that the teacher is not yet ready to give back the test may become irritated at the teacher. Irritation with the teacher can also arouse retaliatory fantasies that can distress the student.

Students were led to believe that exams would be returned on a specified date. This date was pushed back in order to give the teacher more time with the material. Although frustrated, students understood the teacher's stated rationale that more time was needed for grading in order to ensure appropriate attention to the exams.

However, when the teacher was again late returning the exams, several students expressed concern over the implications of the lateness for their ability to prepare adequately for an upcoming examination. A few students were quite angry with the teacher's lateness. The teacher minimized their concern, however, made a comment that the wish for "demand feeding" needed to be curtailed, and stated that grades would be returned in "due time, probably next week." No alteration in the next examination date, two weeks away, was made to accommodate what students felt was the late return of exams.

When the exams were finally returned the following week, one student questioned the teacher after class about whether the grades received were in any way related to students' expressing of feelings about the delay in receiving grades. This was a bold move on the part of the student, who claimed that other students had similar concerns. The teacher was caught off guard by the intensity of these comments and responded in a defensive manner. The teacher claimed to be offended that the student would make such an allegation and suggested that students were externalizing their insecurities. The teacher's comment left the student feeling anxious about the implications that the teacher's obvious resistance could have for the final examination and decided not to pursue the issue further. The entire experience, however, tainted the student's perception of the teacher and of the course.

In this example, the sensitivity of students to potential motivations that underlie the teacher's delay in returning graded work is demonstrated. The example also appears to illustrate how a student's direct expression of realistic concerns about the implications of the teacher's ability to return work on time can exacerbate existing conscious anxieties about academic performance and leave the student with a bitter taste about the entirety of the course experience.

A Comfortable Physical Setting

The quality of the classroom experience is enhanced by a physical setting that is ventilated, lighted, temperate in climate, and spacious. If any of these conditions falls short, students and teacher will feel uncomfortable for the duration of the course. For instance, classrooms that are stuffy, have lights missing, are unseasonably hot or cold, or do not provide chairs and desks for all students convey a message about the value that an institution places on creating a reasonably nurturant physical space within which to do the work of the course.

Under such conditions, students may feel cramped or chilled. Unpleasant somatic sensations color motivations to attend class, listen attentively, and participate. It is often the teacher who must deal with direct questions pertaining to a student's physical comfort in the class. On

the other hand, rooms that are orderly, clean, and comfortable set a tone for students that is inviting.

A group of students were taking a course in a classroom
that had poor ventilation. No comment was made about
the ventilation until a point had been reached in the
course when students began to anticipate a final examination. During a discussion, one student mentioned the
almost claustrophobic nature of the room, with specific
reference to the ventilation. Other students then
opened up and commented on other aspects of the
physical environment.

The teacher reacted on two levels; first, by supporting
the manifest complaint and second, by suggesting that
the complaint itself had arisen symptomatically in response to the anxiety associated with the pending examination. That is, the anxiety about the examination
had sensitized one student to the claustrophobic quality
of the room and other students to different features of
the physical environment, which were also described in
a less than ideal light.

Students appeared to accept this interpretation and
were able to discuss feelings about the examination.
They also brought to the teacher's attention real concerns about the physical setup of the classroom, which
may have contributed to their anxiety about the examination as well as being a symptomatic reaction to it.
Appropriate adjustments in the physical setting were
made in response to these concerns.

This example shows how dimensions of the physical
setting of the classroom embody underlying meaning that
can influence a student's sense of being psychically held
by the teacher. The teacher's attentiveness to the physical
aspects of the classroom setting can help to illuminate

other issues with which students are struggling while also indicating the teacher's respect for the reality of their concerns.

Appropriate Limitations on
Student–Teacher Contact

In a society in which the behavior of psychotherapists has come under increasing public scrutiny, it is critical that any behavior threatening the trust of either clients or subordinates be monitored and modified accordingly. In the field of psychotherapy, for example, the need for such rigorous observation of professional behavior is suggested by survey data (Rodolfa et al. 1994) depicting therapists' susceptibility to sexualizing relationships with clients. Beyond self-report data, however, lie the unsettling unconscious meanings that clients attach to what on the surface may appear to be even the most innocuous contacts with therapists. To this end, Smith (1991) provided a vignette to illustrate the manner in which minor boundary violations involving minimal contact between client and therapist can nevertheless stimulate unconscious fantasies of sexual violation in clients.

The issue of what constitutes appropriate physical distance in a professional relationship extends beyond the client–therapist relationship to other professions, including academe. The American Association of University Professors (AAUP) has offered an articulate presentation of the relationship between sexual harassment and academic freedom (Brown et al. 1994) that delineates contemporary issues in the professional obligations of faculty in an academic setting. The academic environment provides several opportunities for regulated contact between teacher and students. For example, students and teacher convene through class, advisement meetings, phone calls related to questions about the course, college-sponsored functions, and professional meetings that serve both teacher and student. The reality of the teacher's evaluative responsibility, however, would seem to preclude any relationship between teacher and student other than that defined by the formality of teacher and student roles.

Given these considerations, the teacher may be well served to abstain from physical contact, recreational socializing, and other types of relating that may arouse unconscious fantasies in students about the teacher's subjectivity, favoritism, and general ability to maintain appropriate boundaries in the academic environment. In the service of maintaining such boundaries, the teacher may find himself or herself in the awkward position of declining well-intentioned social invitations or other off-campus opportunities to convene with students that are neither related to, nor defined by, the roles of teacher and student. Such abstention may at times be difficult for students to understand and may even lead the teacher to question the merit of his or her position should students report feeling distanced by the teacher's actions. Ultimately, however, the decision to refrain from extracurricular contacts with students serves to hold a professorial stance designed to build some safeguards into the integrity of the student's educational experience. By striving to keep appropriate boundaries and not misuse student trust, the teacher not only helps to protect the integrity of the student–teacher relationship, but can serve as a role model in this regard.

A student was impressed by the manner in which a teacher was able to address with sensitivity and perceptiveness a wide range of delicate issues in a class dealing with the dynamics of human relationships. The student, who was in the midst of some personal difficulties, phoned and inquired about beginning psychotherapy with the teacher. The student indicated the need for therapy but did not say much about the nature of the concern. The teacher declined to accept the therapy referral but explained the rationale behind this decision to the student in a manner that was sensitive to the student's disappointment. The teacher referred the student to a professional in the community. Soon thereafter, the student thanked the teacher for the referral, claimed to understand the decision to refer, and reported feeling better since initiating therapy.

This example serves to depict some of the normal tension that exists for both student and teacher around extra-classroom involvements. In this case, the student encountered a teacher who embodied attributes consistent with good therapy skills. Given that a comfort level had been reached through contact in the classroom, the student inquired about beginning therapy with the teacher. The teacher was sensitive to the ethical issues involved in treating a student in psychotherapy and used the student's request as an opportunity to inform the student about ethical considerations and to direct the student toward another professional who could serve a similar helping function. The teacher was thus able to refrain from taking advantage of the student's idealization that had occurred in the classroom and hold to appropriate boundaries between student and teacher.

Respectful Dialogue

The tensions that emerge around learning, not unlike some of the tensions that emerge during the course of psychoanalytic therapy, can create stress in the teacher–student relationship. Respectful dialogue with students involves attentive listening and responses that are thoughtful, ethical, relevant, and facilitative to learning.

Here, the teacher desists from aggressive, sexualized, or other inappropriate modes of dialogue.

A student took umbrage at a comment that a teacher made in class. The comment itself was related to an article that the class had been required to read. In making a comment on the article, the teacher stated that the author had neglected to present a balanced view. Added balance would have emphasized a type of therapy that the teacher favored. The teacher commented that the author's preferred approach, while having merit, also had some limitations, which the teacher then addressed.

However, unbeknownst to the teacher, the student's therapist was an advocate of the approach. The student sought out the teacher before the next class and voiced strong sentiments about the value of the approach recommended in the article. The teacher stated that the comments made in class were in the service of offering a balanced view rather than an indictment of the author's model.

During the early part of their meeting, the teacher had the fantasy of challenging the author's approach more aggressively, but decided against this action and instead listened as the student voiced concern. About ten minutes into the meeting, the student began to relax and actually talked about sharing some of the same misgivings that the teacher had voiced during class. The student was able to see that the teacher's remarks had touched a personal chord. The meeting ended with the student's feeling a deeper appreciation for the teacher's intentions when critiquing the article.

In this example, the teacher's ability to maintain composure while under fire allowed the student to voice concerns and eventually achieve a better understanding of

the teacher's motives. Had the teacher openly returned the
student's anger or challenged the student's personal therapy, the direction of the exchange would have been of
little educational benefit to the student.

Appropriate Fee Structure

Students and faculty contract for a course through the
school. Students pay tuition directly to the school; in turn,
the school is responsible for assuring quality instruction in
the classroom and remunerates accordingly. In some
ways, this arrangement is akin to a managed care process
but with different players. Here the student is the client,
who pays into a system and receives a fixed number of
classes; the teacher is the provider, who works within a
designated salary range set by the school; and the school is
the regulating body that passes final judgment on the
quality of care.

When tuition and remuneration are commensurate with
local standards, both students and faculty experience a
sense of fairness. For students, advance notification and
rationale for tuition increments permit sufficient time for
appropriate budgetary allocation and planning and contribute to a sense of participation in a school's continuing
development as an institution of higher education. Faculty
salaries that are reasonable in light of comparative trends
strengthen faculty unity and spirit. The ability to set and
hold to a reasonable fiscal policy, despite external pressure to modify, can strengthen a school's identity with
both its students and faculty.

A teacher was recruited to teach a specialty course and
agreed to be remunerated in accordance with the policy
for adjunct teaching. Soon after the semester began, the
teacher began to complain openly about the remuneration. Several students informed an administrator that
the teacher had voiced complaints about salary during

class. The students feared that the teacher's attitude was detrimental to the class and asked the administrator to intervene.

The administrator weighed various alternatives and decided to contact the teacher in order to find out how the course was going. Reluctant to state that students had expressed their concerns in a private meeting, the administrator hoped that the teacher would spontaneously express feelings about the salary issue. Within moments of initiating conversation, the teacher spoke openly about the salary concern and asked for an adjustment in salary. The teacher also stated that the concern about the amount of money being paid had actually come up in class. The teacher felt remorse about this disclosure to the class and wondered if students had commented about this issue to the administrator. The administrator then informed the teacher about having had a brief contact with students during which they voiced concern about the teacher's remarks.

What followed was an open discussion about the teacher's feelings. Both the teacher and the administrator felt relieved that they had been able to discuss the issue without either party's becoming angered to the point that student welfare might be compromised. They considered the implications of raising the teacher's salary, but decided that to raise the salary of one teacher would be potentially divisive for all faculty, if and when other faculty became aware of this modification. Furthermore, initial negotiations had occurred in good faith; to break the contract would create administrative problems that could resonate to other organizational levels. The teacher agreed to continue to teach at the original salary, and no further remarks about remunerative inequity were discussed with students in class.

In this example, the ability of an administrator to listen to all concerned parties, to consider the deliberate risks and advantages of modifying an arrangement made in good faith, and to reflect on implications for the classroom and for the entire administrative system helped to defuse a potentially volatile situation. For example, harsh criticism of the teacher's sense of professionalism may have alienated the teacher and not served the concerns of students. On the other hand, yielding to the teacher's request for more money would have had the equally deleterious impact of alienating other faculty while offering no promise that the teacher who had requested the increase in salary would have been assuaged by the granting of this request.

Relative Confidentiality

Total confidentiality in the academic setting is an impossibility. Student files contain reference letters, grades, and other pertinent information that is made available to faculty who have admitting and evaluative responsibilities in a program of study. It is possible, however, within the limitations of the educational setting, to afford students relative confidentiality.

Relative confidentiality refers to holding in confidence personal material about a student that is deemed to be outside the scope of formal institutional review. Included here is material that may have been presented to a faculty member in another context outside the school, such as during a supervisory relationship that predated either the student's or the faculty member's involvement with the school. In this situation, a student may have divulged personal material to the faculty member when the faculty member was a work supervisor. The public revelation of this material in the academic setting, however, would be inappropriate.

A second source of such information may be unsolicited material presented by a student to a faculty member because of the faculty member's perceived integrity. Such material may include a student's divulging a concern about another student to the faculty member. For instance, one student may voice concern about what the student perceives to be another student's emotional problems. In this case, the faculty member listens and may inquire about the quality of relationship between the two students, but would be hard pressed to approach the person about whom the student is concerned without risking grievous consequences for the relationship between the student and this person, the faculty member and the person, the faculty member and the student, and the program as a whole.

Prior to entering a graduate program, a student had been supervised at work by a faculty member. The supervision had occurred several years before the faculty member started teaching in the program. Personal material had been divulged by the student during supervision in the context of better understanding countertransference reactions to a certain client.

While this student was taking a course from the faculty member, clinical material was presented by another student that was very similar to the clinical material on which the first student had been supervised. The student had an uneasy moment and wondered if the teacher would reference the supervisory relationship or even look at the student in a way that would exacerbate the student's already heightened level of self-consciousness. The teacher did not say or do anything that would have made the student squirm. After class, the student approached the teacher ostensibly about another issue in the course, but wondered if the teacher would in any way acknowledge the meaning of the clinical material under discussion in class as it pertained to their supervisory work. Much to the student's surprise and delight, the teacher said nothing about their supervisory relationship.

This example highlights the sensitivity that students have to material that is offered in confidence and has no tangible role in the academic evaluation process. Faculty members who are able to make distinctions along these lines provide students with a measure of relief and a source of strength during potentially tenuous moments in an academic setting.

Formal Course Evaluation By Students

Much in the same way that psychotherapy clients engage in ongoing assessment, both consciously and unconsciously, of the quality of their therapists' work, so too do students continually assess the quality of their teachers' performance. Such assessment of teachers by students is almost exclusively of a private, internal nature, save for the formal, written course evaluations that institutions require. Course evaluations are usually handled at the end of a course.

Course evaluations provide students with the opportunity to evaluate anonymously the quality of teaching, the interpersonal atmosphere of the class, and the usefulness of the course within the context of the curriculum. These evaluations are also vehicles of communication between students and academic administrators. In addition to quantitative assessment, course evaluations may contain qualitative commentary that casts faculty members in favorable or unfavorable light. Without access to evaluations, administrators may be unable to document faculty teaching performance from the perspective of the students whom they teach. Quality of teaching performance may be a determining factor in faculty promotion. The implications of course evaluations thus resonate not only for students but also for faculty members.

One way to orchestrate the evaluation procedure and keep it as private as possible is to create psychological safety for students around the entirety of the evaluation experience. Under ideal circumstances, this aim may entail conducting the evaluations during class time but with the faculty member not present in the room. Evaluations may then be placed in an envelope, sealed, and returned to the appropriate administrative personnel by a student. The evaluations are kept in a private file until such time as they can be made accessible to faculty. Faculty are not given access to these evaluations until after the course has been completed and all grades have been determined. Students should be informed of this procedure as a way of safeguarding their freedom to evaluate so that conscious and unconscious fears of retribution that arise in the context of evaluating the performance of a faculty member do not become magnified. Failure to follow any of the steps in this protocol may arouse a heightened sense of vulnerability for students and faculty.

> Evaluations were distributed to a class and were turned in to the central office in accordance with appropriate procedure. Evaluations were tabulated in an open setting, however, with several individuals having access to the content of the evaluations. A faculty member noticed this oversight and raised protest around the need to protect the privacy of both students and faculty during the evaluation process. This complaint was addressed promptly, and additional steps were taken to ensure high levels of security for public displays of course evaluations.

This example appears to illustrate the sensitivity of faculty to being evaluated and the necessity of establishing a protective, private environment around the entire evaluation process. Such privacy not only affords students additional psychological support when they evaluate their faculty, but also displays sensitivity to the self-esteem issues aroused for faculty when they are evaluated by their students.

CHAPTER 5

Student–Teacher Dynamics and Intrapsychic Processes: Psychosexuality, Ego Functions, Object Relations, and Selfobject Needs

The dynamic interplay between student and teacher that unfolds within the teaching framework is at the hub of the classroom environment. The unique personal histories that student and teacher bring to the classroom color the perceptions that make their interactions meaningful. The richness and texture of these interactions shape much of what defines academic life—quality of instruction, sentiment about faculty, institutional reputation, commitment to learning and to service—the list goes on and on.

In the classroom, the psychoanalytic educator has a veritable gold mine from which to extract insights into the types of relationships that make higher education so unique in this culture. For it is within the academic environment, especially within the classroom, that seeds of professional knowledge, professional identity, and sense of service that will guide the clinical student for years to come are sown. But the psychoanalytically informed educator also faces many challenges when seeking to apply psychoanalytic theory to classroom observation. Operating within a relatively defined theoretical framework, the teacher must draw on the analytic literature in order to understand what makes the individual psychologies of teacher and student come alive in the classroom. In some ways, the challenges facing a teacher of analytic persuasion are not that different from those confronting the contemporary psychoanalytic practitioner.

Over the years, creative thinkers have introduced supple analytic constructs that have stood the test of time. From psychosexuality to self psychology, analytic theory has been blessed with metaphors that offer plausible explanations of the human condition. Recently, such analytic writers as Greenberg and Mitchell (1983), Mitchell (1993), Pine (1990), Pulver (1993), and Schafer (1992) have discussed how different models within analytic theory each have something of value to say about personality dynamics and the relationship between client and therapist. Each model offers a perspective, a way of viewing the client's internal world, that, within the context of relativism, is as meaningful as the next. Perhaps Lerner (1994) best summed up the merit of taking an open-minded, integrative stance in relation to different analytic theories when he stated:

I have long considered myself a nonclassical analyst with leanings toward an object relations point of view. This comes from the recognition that psychoanalysis is not a monolithic, well-integrated theory, but rather a loose composite of various submodels. It has been my experience that each of the submodels—drive theory, structural theory, self theory and object relations theory—has something to contribute to our understanding of patients. [p. 573]

Clearly it would appear that a positive development in psychoanalytic theory is its movement toward a new synthesis of ideas. As an applied discipline, psychoanalytic education benefits from developments dictated by the expansion of theory and technique. One task for the psychoanalytic educator would therefore seem to involve drawing on a range of concepts that can maximize potential understandings of phenomena between students and teachers at a given point in time.

In this chapter, I draw on four theoretical concepts that remain vital to an analytic understanding of intrapsychic life and apply them to the classroom situation. These concepts—psychosexuality, ego functions, self and object representations, and selfobject needs—which derive respectively from drive theory, ego psychology, object relations theory, and self psychology, help to capture the internal worlds of teacher and student as these worlds are portrayed psychoanalytically. In isolation, each concept serves as a central organizer for a theoretical base within psychoanalytic-educational psychology. Together, however, they can be understood to represent different aspects of a unitary psychic phenomenon. Pine (1990) has discussed the constructs of drive, ego, object relations, and self as being critical to our understanding of the totality of intrapsychic life. Each of these four constructs has something unique and valuable to add to an understanding of the classroom setting.

PSYCHOSEXUALITY

Included among Freud's writings (Rychlak 1973) are his ideas about infantile sexuality and the psychosexual stages of development. Freud's ideas about psychosexuality serve as a series of organizing constructs for the development of pathological character trends. Not only is psychosexuality a prime topic among analytic theoreticians, but its implications have also been integrated into middle-class colloquialism applied to personality. It is not unusual, for example, to locate such terms as *oral needs, anal character*, and *oedipal conflict* in literary or cinematic references to psychological functioning of protagonists. Moreover, rare is the abnormal psychology text that does not pay some attention to sexual instincts, their normal path of maturation, and implications for everyday psychopathology.

Psychosexuality is thought to have as its basis the tension between sexual and aggressive instinctual drives and social prohibitions against their expression. As a biological model of psychological functioning, Freud envisioned an intimate relationship between mind and body in which primal instincts shape the development of intrapsychic structures, which in turn shape the objects of the external world. Intrapsychic development is now thought to be heavily influenced by the quality of a child's experiences associated with particular bodily sensations in the oral, anal, and genital zones. That is, adult development inevitably reflects the way in which the child navigated psychological tasks related to these different bodily zones.

This proposition is at once both intriguing and inviting to the studied observer of child development. It is inviting insofar as it provides a broad-based fit between retrospective deductions from present level of functioning to early childhood conflict. Yet it remains open to considerable debate precisely because of the experience-distant terminology on which it stands. Indeed, Freud's choice of an experience-distant language that is both abstruse and intangible has proven costly to psychoanalytic psychology's effort to be received as a humanistic psychology within professional circles, despite Bettelheim's (1982) eloquent request for a reappraisal of Freud's writings in their original tongue.

Psychosexuality and the Psychoanalytic Educator

An inescapable necessity for the psychoanalytic educator is the classroom challenge of helping students discover the wisdom in Freud's writings without becoming bogged down in endless dialogue concerning the veracity of mechanistic terminology. How can Freud's psychosexual idiom be translated in a way that informs the teacher about the vicissitudes of the classroom? More specifically, how can the psychosexual paradigm inform the classroom process?

Sutherland's Psychosexuality Model for Learning Stages

Sutherland (1951) offered a developmental stage model of the learning process for medical students that draws on Freud's model of psychosexuality and is applicable to clinical training in mental health. Building on Freud's model, Sutherland presented a series of inevitable points of tension in the learning process that were characterized by the students' playing out in adulthood vestiges of infantile psychosexuality as part of a developmental progression toward higher levels of competence and self-confidence.

The earliest stage of training is marked by the students' assuming the position of passive learners, who need teachers to supply and sustain knowledge acquisition and maturation. In this stage, teachers are presumed to be readily available to produce knowledge for students on demand. The manner in which students present during the earliest phases of training is offered as a corollary to the early infantile stage of oral passivity when the infant uses the mother's availability to orient to, and absorb, the external world as presented through the timeliness and quality of the mother's ministrations.

From this early stage, students then move, metaphorically, to a more active orality, with a higher level of inquisitiveness and more participation in the learning process. In this phase, teachers may feel pressure to give more supplies as students press for more knowledge, although they still enact this demand primarily through a dependent position.

Normal developmental progression as a learner next leads the student into an analog of the anal phase, when independent strivings and a desire to carve personalized learning interests conflict with pressure to continue to conform to what may now be perceived as the rather rigid nature of the fixed curriculum. In this stage, students may feel that their autonomous striving as learners is being squelched by basic course requirements. Defiance of such perceived conformity demands may find expression in coming late to class, leaving class early, and perfunctorily completing parts of the curriculum.

It is here, too, that first-time power struggles may emerge in the relationship between teacher and students. One may infer, for example, a situation in which students have begun to feel more comfortable taking risks through the independent manipulation of constructs. Such independence may be evidenced through creative displays in which students begin to feel familiar with constructs that were previously difficult to comprehend and start to synthesize ideas in new ways. Because students are on new ground, there may be a special vulnerability to the anal-based fantasies of embarrassment or humiliation at the hands of the teacher-authority.

As students progress beyond this stage, they move easily into a phase of development similar to the phallic-urethral stage when creative displays of knowledge and mature assertion take firm hold. Under less optimal conditions, students who had earlier requested supplies from the teacher and had shown some defiance around the teacher's request for conformity may now belittle the teacher's expertise. In either case, students may feel competitive with each other, but at the same time seek to forge alliances among themselves in response to perceptions of authority as attempting to minimize their self-assertion. In this phase, the teacher may experience challenges to his or her most cherished beliefs and must be mindful of the necessity of giving students space to find their own niche within the learning environment.

During the final stage of development in the learning process, which is portrayed as being symbolic of the genital phase of psychosexuality, students move toward collegial, competitive positions with faculty and, in turn, may develop realistic appraisals of professional life as seen from the perspective of a faculty member. There is less of a concern both with challenging and being accepted by faculty and more of an investment in synthesizing their own thoughts. Strongly toned affective reactions to faculty diminish as formal course work ends and students move closer to program completion.

The value of this type of psychoanalytic-educational model is that it describes the intrapsychic dynamics of students in a manner sensitive to drives, development, atypicality, and phenomenology. Students can be tracked through the educational process, and their development can be monitored through application of a theory such as the one proposed by Sutherland.

EGO FUNCTIONS

The delineation of the concept of the ego and its various functions represented an advance in psychoanalytic theory. This advancement was marked by moving the ego away from its original position as an extension of, and conduit for, the raw, id-based drives and toward a comprehensive psychology in which the ego is given a distinctive role in fostering attachment to the environment. Rather than subordinated to the id, the ego was described by Hartmann (1958) as representing the innate, unfolding, autonomous capacities of the organism nestled within a conflict-free sphere of psychic life that facilitates adaptation by regulating drives in response to appropriate environmental stimulation.

Ego psychology provided the analytic theorist with new language for conceptualizing adaptation and psychopathology. Bellak (1975) enumerated as ego functions the following constructs: reality testing; judgment; sense of the world and of the self; regulation and control of drives, affects, and impulses; object relations; thought processes; adaptive regression in the service of the ego; defensive functioning; autonomous functioning; synthetic-integrative functioning; and mastery-competence.

The student–teacher exchange places a premium on ego strength and the balance of ego functions. Mastering course material requires well-developed concept formation, memory, judgment, planning, capacity for delay, and creativity. It also requires appropriate management of affects and impulses in response to internalized object relational paradigms aroused by teacher and student roles.

SELF AND OBJECT REPRESENTATIONS

Within psychoanalytic theory, the construct of object relations is omnipresent. Despite nuances across different theoretical conceptions of object relations (Bellak 1975, Fairbairn 1963, Greenberg and Mitchell 1983, Klein 1975, Mahler et al. 1975), its value as an explanatory construct for intrapsychic life remains indisputable. Internal representations of self and object that become increasingly differentiated foster mature relationships characterized by the ability to appreciate self and others as separate psychological entities.

The capacity for whole object relations and the presence of psychological features that define whole object relations, including mature empathy, mature intimacy, stable identity, and good reality testing, are prerequisite to an optimal educational experience. For example, students and teachers whose internalized object relations are predominantly whole are likely to bring clear interpersonal boundaries, ethicality, cooperation, positive emotions, consideration, and empathy to the classroom and to their relationships with each other. Such maturity allows for appropriate discharge of the types of normal frustrations that emerge during the course of intensive academic study, in a way that raises awareness without provoking anxiety-ridden behaviors in either student or teacher. Moreover, the reality testing that governs these relationships helps protect students and teachers from the prolonged, regressive swings characterized by unstable internal representations that may otherwise make the educational process unproductive.

SELFOBJECT NEEDS

The notion of selfobject needs is born from self psychology. Self psychology (Baker and Baker 1987, Kohut 1971, 1977) has emphasized the role of significant others as selfobjects whose primary function it is to help the youngster develop a cohesive sense of self through the provision of empathic responsiveness. Empathic parental responsiveness is directed toward the psychic needs of the youngster, including (1) mirroring needs—needing to be affirmed and prized, (2) idealizing needs—needing to be soothed by a strong other, and (3) twinship needs—needing to feel a common bond with others.

From a self psychological perspective, inconsistent parental affirmation and erratic patterns of parental soothing or outcasting arouse psychological vulnerability that undergirds the interpersonal and self-regulating difficulties of individuals experiencing distress. In distinguishing self psychology from other psychoanalytic models of intrapsychic life, it is the development of the three selfobject needs in response to empathic responding that identifies mature psychological adaptation.

An additional distinguishing feature of self psychology is the reality-based quality of the parental response. Successes or failures in empathy are rooted in real events and are not fantasized distortions driven by sexualized longings or aggressive tensions. Empathic failures may lead to the sexual or aggressive nature of symptom formation but are not caused by the drives themselves.

The self psychology literature on psychopathology and psychotherapy provides referents for understanding that unfulfilled selfobject needs can find expression in the classroom setting. Empathic failures, poorly integrated exhibitionistic strivings, hypersensitivity to flaws in others, and a sense of being different from others are manifestations of immature selfobject needs.

Connors (1994) has provided a framework for understanding symptom formation from a self psychological perspective that offers insight into some intrapsychic issues that can be cumbersome to students or teachers. Connors suggested that inhibition in patients, for example, can be explained in part by a fear of being overstimulated by grandiose strivings. Rather than move ahead, these patients preserve primitive selfobject bonds to parental figures by sacrificing initiative instead of risking harsh rebuke associated with self-strivings. In the classroom, such sacrifice of initiative may take the form of academic underachievement, whereby the student performs at a level below expected potential.

A similar analogy may be drawn between the fear of

fragmenting that characterizes the anxious, avoidant, or phobic patient and the types of behaviors that may severely compromise a student's performance in specific academic situations. For instance, students who have problems managing anxiety during tests, who never talk in class, who become extremely self-conscious during presentations, or who attend class only erratically can be understood within a self psychological paradigm as having difficulty regulating self-esteem. The origin of the self-esteem vulnerability is rooted in real empathic failure. The anticipation of again being subjected to harshness, overstimulation, indifference, or alienation can be strong enough to squelch mature strivings and to interfere with school performance.

The emergence of unmet selfobject needs in teachers can also take different shapes. Manifestations include abuses of power issuing from the teacher's need to be admired, grade inflation issuing from the teacher's fear of alienating students, and self-serving displays issuing from the teacher's need for affirmation, which overstimulates students and creates discomfort in the classroom.

Self psychology offers insight into the ebbs and flows of mentoring relationships between teachers and students. Students' needs to feel affirmed, safe, and bonded in relation to their teachers are normal needs that students bring to the academic setting. Similarly, teachers need to feel prized, admired, and bonded with their students. When these needs are exaggerated, however, the potential for problems multiplies (Cozzarrelli and Silin 1989).

Mehlman and Glickauf-Hughes (1994) examined the way in which disturbances in selfobject needs stress the mentoring relationship. They focused on the activation of idealizing, mirroring, and twinship needs in both students and teachers in the context of the intense relationships that students and teachers form. A student with strong needs to idealize a teacher may strike up an intense attachment only to become disillusioned should the professor fail to meet the unusually high standards set by the student. On the other hand, a teacher with a strong need to be idealized may foster dependency attachments with students in order to stabilize his or her own self-esteem.

In cases where the student has a strong need for affirmation, there may be problems hearing the constructive aspects of feedback, requests for affirmation of uniqueness, or sensitivity to being slighted that takes a subtle form, such as feeling ignored if another student is called on to answer a question. Similarly, the teacher who has a strong mirroring need may, for example, have difficulty identifying exceptional work by students because of conflicts associated with the grandiose sector of his or her own personality.

When twinship needs are prominent, the student attaches himself or herself to a mentor who is perceived by the student to share a work ethic, level of sensitivity, or interest in a specific topic. Often there is a mind-reading fantasy in which perceived similarity of interest precludes verbalizing thoughts and feelings. For instance, the student may feel that there is no need to clear a term paper topic with the teacher, despite a request that all class members do so, because the student assumes that the teacher "knows what I want to do it on." Under these conditions, opportunity for misperception is intensified. Gradual awareness of real differences with the teacher can therefore be quite painful for the student with strong twinship needs. To this end, teachers who wish to spawn protégés or proselytes may have problems accepting the maturation of a student's interest in a direction other than that sanctioned by the teacher. Or the teacher may struggle with the desire to turn teaching relationships into friendships, prematurely viewing students as colleagues, and seeking to engage them on a social level that brings the possibility of dual roles into the relationship.

CLINICAL MATERIAL

A student was planning to present a clinical case in a seminar. It was to be the student's first such presentation. For weeks prior to the scheduled presentation, the student noticed a gradual increase in anticipatory anxiety and began to vacillate about which case to present to the seminar group and the teacher, whom the student admired. The student's indecision centered around the presentation of an easy case versus a more challenging case. The former case would probably not invite much critique; the latter case would expose more of the student's skill limitations but also held the promise of inviting valuable feedback.

In deliberating this issue, the student was aware that the tenor of the seminar was very supportive, although there were times during class when it appeared to the student that class members tried to outdo each other when offering inferences about the cases that were being reviewed. It was the student's impression that the seminar leader encouraged students to speak their mind and did not stifle open discussion, but that students depended on the seminar leader to actually give the "right" answer whenever the level of questioning raised several alternative answers.

The student thought that this type of format was of value precisely because it fostered the sharing of ideas in a supportive atmosphere. Yet this same impression also made the student anxious because it conjured up images of the student's own family of origin in which the student's mother appeared to openly encourage competition among her children. The student had fantasies of the seminar leader's stepping in and assuaging any potential anxiety arising during the presentation. The student also had recall, however, of an incident when the seminar leader was perceived as aggressive in chal-

lenging another student; the recollection of this incident on the eve of the student's own presentation made
the student anxious.

On the day of the presentation, the student selected
the harder case but began the presentation by fumbling
the few papers on which case notes had been scrawled.
There was a momentary heightening of self-consciousness that was followed by the student's summary of the
course of treatment. This summary was punctuated by
the student's asking seminar members if they had questions; all such requests were met by silence.

The student then presented a specific session after
which seminar members began to discuss the case. The
student was able to field questions in a thoughtful
manner and talked in a genuine tone about countertransference dilemmas. Other students in the seminar
were supportive and insightful. One student even noted
that at one point during a reading of the case, the
presenter had two reading miscues. A very lively discussion ensued about countertransference implications.
The presenter also questioned the client's diagnosis in
light of what had been learned in this particular class. In
general, seminar members were quick to agree with
each other's impressions of the case.

The seminar leader had remained silent until near the
end of the seminar, when the student asked, "What are
your impressions of the case?" The leader responded by
praising the student's effort to work with a difficult
client and the quality of class dialogue that developed
around the case. The seminar leader then self-disclosed
about having worked with a similar client when in
training and drew on this experience to assist the class
in understanding the client's psychopathology. Examples of how to respond to the client's pressing concerns
were also offered. The presenter then spontaneously
disclosed other case material, related to a second client

who was also difficult to treat, in which a critical maternal figure had been supplanted by a positive role model at a decisive juncture in the client's maturation into young adulthood. The presenter was able to identify similarities between the first and second clients in a way that had not been noted previously. At this point, the seminar ended.

ANALYSIS: STUDENT DYNAMICS

Psychosexuality: Applicability of Sutherland's Model

The presenter's behavior appears to be consistent with Sutherland's phase of active orality. Active orality as a learning stage within a psychosexual model of the educational process is characterized by the student's inquisitiveness, active participation in the learning process, and dependency, as well as by the teacher's felt pressure to supply the student with encouragement and immediate feedback.

In the present case, the student's inquisitiveness was manifested by the internal dilemma about which case to share with the group. The student was thoughtful, deliberated the pros and cons of sharing different cases, eventually decided on the more challenging case, and displayed curiosity about how to understand both countertransference reactions and the client's psychopathology in relation to what the student had been taught in class. The type of dependency that characterizes this phase is denoted by the student's anxiously asking the teacher for direct feedback.

Ego Functioning

Disruptions in ego functioning can be understood in relation to the infiltration of drive material into different ego domains. For example, slippage in motoric or perceptual functioning, inefficiency in decision making, defensive fantasy, and subtle reality distortions all signal disturbance in ego functioning. In the present case, mild disruptions in the student's ego functioning are suggested by the brief indecision about which case to present, fantasies of being protected by the teacher from critical review by classmates (who, in turn, may have been displacement objects in response to fantasized rebuke by the teacher–maternal figure), fumbling with papers, reading miscues, and elevated self-consciousness (and heightening of projective defenses) when requests for questions were met by silence.

Adaptive functioning appears to be reflected by the student's ability to seek the teacher's support and insight. Other indications of adaptive ego functioning seem to occur in response to the presence of two supportive interpersonal measures. Here the active involvement of classmates during the case discussion and the teacher's supportive praise and advice appear associated with the attenuation of the anxiety-evoking quality of the student's internalized representations and the higher-level synthesis of the case material.

Object Relations

From an object-relational perspective, the student's internalized object representations include an image of self as vulnerable and an image of the maternal figure as encouraging aggression in her offspring by adopting a slow-to-protect attitude in situations that heightened competitive tensions. It may be argued that the arousal of this particular paradigm in the context of the seminar shaped the student's anticipatory anxiety about the presentation. The level of object relatedness, however, appears to be whole. Whole object relations are evidenced by the ambivalency that characterizes the student's reaction to the seminar leader. Such ambivalency is indicative of whole object relatedness because it reflects the capacity to hold both positive and negative affect states simultaneously in relation to a significant other. There was, for instance, a desire to please the teacher, which did not cancel out the anger associated with the fantasy that the teacher might not protect the student should the student feel vulnerable during the presentation. Instead, both affect states were present and directed toward a single person in a way that reflects whole object relations. Symptomatic expression of the student's vulnerability was present and included fumbling with papers, reading miscues, and self-consciousness.

From the object-relational perspective, the fantasized withdrawal of maternal supplies would be considered the primary determinant of the student's symptomatic reaction. The student's anxious query to the teacher about the quality of the presentation appears to reflect a fantasy that the teacher had withdrawn support at a point when the student needed the teacher's availability. The teacher was appropriately responsive to this request, and the presentation ended with highly organized functioning.

Selfobject Needs

The self psychological position would understand the presenter's symptomatic reactions as being secondary to an anticipated diminution of a selfobject bond with the teacher. The student admired the teacher and may have feared that the teacher would not be able to calm whatever anxiety was aroused by the presentation. There was also a fear that praise might not be forthcoming in response to having accomplished the presentation. In addition, the anticipation of small fractures in bonds with classmates also factored into the presenter's anxiety. These three concerns seem organized around, respectively, idealizing, mirroring, and twinning needs. Symptomatic reactions during the presentation appear to signal a decrease in the cohesion of self experience. These reactions led the presenter to seek direct support from the teacher. The teacher's response was experienced empathically as evidenced by the positive imagery depicting another client's progress that emerged following the teacher's comments. Such imagery can be taken as a reflection of the presenter's having felt strengthened by the teacher's supportive, empathic remarks.

ANALYSIS: TEACHER DYNAMICS

The teacher's intrapsychic dynamics color all aspects of the teacher's experience at a given point in time. The degree to which the teacher struggles with dependency, control, and competitive issues or is desirous or fearful of being affirmed or idealized serves to mediate various reactions to students. Ideally, the teacher is relatively unencumbered by such conflicts in the learning situation, with formulation and intervention based almost exclusively on accurate perceptions of student need.

Formulations derive from an understanding of the ways such constructs as psychosexuality, ego functions, self and object representations, and selfobject needs impact the intrapsychic dynamics of students. Some questions may help the teacher understand student dynamics. Is the student angered, anxious, or pressured? Does the student see self as a victim or a victimizer? Is the student anticipating danger or affirmation? How settled is the student's performance? Does the student seem at ease or disjointed? How do others seem to be reacting to the student? Are they engaged? Tense? Dispirited?

Teacher interventions issue from the way in which student dynamics impact the teacher. When the teacher is in reasonable psychological balance, interventions should be empathic, explanatory, and useful. Students who are in the beginning phases of training may, for example, require direct support and encouragement in order to cope with a stressful moment, whereas more advanced and self-confident students need room to challenge each other and the teacher as a way of forging a higher synthesis of material.

In the present example, the teacher appears to have been sensitive to the student's developmental position and provided a supportive yet instructive comment as a way of nurturing the student's self-confidence. Had the teacher's own conflicts around dependency, idealization, mirroring, or competition been aroused to an uncomfortable level in response to the student's request for direct feedback, then the response would have been different and potentially too strong to benefit the student. This interpretation seems to be most consistent with the value of responding to the student's selfobject need for affirmation.

Using drive theory as a point of contrast, one can argue that the teacher's supportive comment did not permit exploration of the student's fear of not having handled the case well. Maybe the teacher was angry with the student and defended against this anger with a reaction-formation that minimized any expression of anger through the supportive remark. In addition, the teacher's self-disclosure may be interpreted as embodying a mild competitive element. The competitive element is evidenced by the teacher's need to make clear to the student that the teacher was far beyond the type of dilemma that the student was now confronting as a beginning therapist. The teacher's need to self-disclose may be understood here as reflecting first an unconscious identification with the vulnerable student and then a defense against the attraction of this identification through a mildly exhibitionistic-competitive display that may be reflective of phallic-exhibitionistic issues.

DISCUSSION

Because no one person can serve as his or her own control in an exacting sense, it is impossible to determine whether a different teacher intervention phrased with different emphases to a different student would have produced the same type of student response as did the intervention posed by the teacher in the clinical example. Thus, it is impossible to determine whether a nondirective comment around the student's request for support, or an interpretive comment helping the student appreciate that the request for support was an adaptive effort to stave off an underlying anxiety perhaps paralleling the client's experience, would have been received empathically by the student at that moment in the presentation. Any number of plausible venues can be pursued in response to any given student. For a teacher's intervention to be of use to a student, however, it needs to be empathic, explanatory, and facilitative to learning. Such a teaching intervention, much like a good therapeutic intervention, remains sensitive to dimensions of experience captured by the constructs of drives, ego functions, self and object representations, and selfobject needs. Each idea adds to an understanding of the intrapsychic processes of teacher and student.

CHAPTER 6

Student–Teacher Dynamics and Interpersonal Processes: Transference, Countertransference, and Projective Identification

Classroom interaction is continuous. Student and teacher communicate with each other directly, through questions and answers; indirectly, through selection of term paper topics and spontaneous disclosure of case material; and nonverbally, through various forms of behavioral gesturing that allows discharge of tension in class. Indeed, amid the dialogue that accompanies the manifest course content, there are many other dialogues going on between teacher and student.

Three psychoanalytically derived interpersonal processes help to explain the communication of intrapsychic contents governing transactions between teacher and student. These three processes—transference, countertransference, and projective identification—which embody intrapsychic substrata, are central to any psychoanalytic understanding of interpersonal communications. Both the intrapsychic and interpersonal perspectives on psychological functioning inform our experiences of human discourse, including interactions between student and teacher.

THE INTERPERSONAL DIMENSION OF
EXPERIENCE

Before presenting a review and classroom application of the concepts of transference, countertransference, and projective identification, I think it is helpful to provide a rationale for my identification of intrapsychic and interpersonal considerations as being different enough from each other to warrant separate attention. By distinguishing intrapsychic and interpersonal dimensions of experience, I do not mean to imply a definitive separation between these two domains. Rather, I view them as two aspects of a unitary psychological experience, with sufficient differentiation to warrant separate identities, but sufficient overlap to acknowledge commonality.

On a continuum, interpersonal events can be depicted as emanating from diverse origins. For example, an interpersonal event can seemingly exist in one person's fantasy, such as when one person has thoughts about another person who is unaware of being an object of a fantasy. There can also be a more active delivery of one person's intrapsychic content into another person, such as when one person's fantasy begins to encroach on the psychology of the other person, who then begins to react to this fantasy material by identifying with it. This identification may be accompanied by an active response to the fantasy, such that relational pressure is now directed back toward the other person in a way that revises the quality of interaction. Or there may be a passive response to this same material in which silent reflection, rather than overt behavioral response, including forceful projection, is dominant. The line between intrapsychic and interpersonal dynamics is continuous and discernible, but fine.

A student hesitates for a moment to raise his hand when the teacher asks the class for an answer to a question. It goes up only partially, then is anxiously pulled down, then shoots up again, but by then it is too late. Another student beats him to the punch, puts her hand up first, is called on by the teacher, and then gives the same correct answer that the cautious student would have given had he been a bit more confident in his ability to deliver a correct response.

The student who was slow to raise his hand reacts by visibly slumping in his seat while nodding his head in agreement with the correct answer. Both movements do not escape the teacher's eye. The teacher reacts viscerally and cognitively to the student's nonverbal gesturing by sensing that the student feels as if he had lost an opportunity to show the teacher and his classmates what he could do and by speculating silently about the motivations and meanings underlying the student's behavior.

In this example, the student's conscious and unconscious reasons for momentarily hesitating to raise his hand at that moment with that teacher in that class can be understood as having both intrapsychic and interactional dimensions. With an intrapsychic focus, one may argue that the student was afraid of the consequences of possibly being wrong in the eyes of the teacher and his classmates. Such consequences may include, for example, the fantasy that, if wrong, there may be insensitivity to effort, silent ridicule by teacher or peers, overstimulation of self as inadequate, or whatever other meanings the student may attach to the event. Or the student may have feared the consequence of being the first one with the correct answer. This fear, too, may have triggered an anxious fantasy constellation but of a different sort, possibly an anxious retreat from what may have been defined as a competitive moment in which the student saw himself as being in a position to outshine others.

In either instance, the student's momentary ambivalence about raising his hand can be conceptualized as a way of protecting himself from the conflictual implications of being called on by the teacher. Although these implications occurred intrapsychically, they nonetheless became imbued with interpersonal meanings in the context of the student's intrapsychic life. A second and more obvious way to conceptualize the interpersonal dimension of this experience can be drawn from the student's nonverbal behavior. It was the student's nonverbal actions that appeared to heighten the teacher's experience of the student's presence in class such that the teacher began to think and feel differently about the nuances of the aforementioned events.

The intrapsychic and interpersonal dimensions of experience are closely related, although from a clinical standpoint we recognize them as different aspects of the human condition. Gill (1982) has cogently described the merit of not thinking about intrapsychic and interpersonal processes dichotomously, but rather as intertwined in the fabric of interpersonal relations. The interpersonal processes that communicate intrapsychic content are the psychoanalytic phenomena of transference, countertransference, and projective identification, each of which is applicable to the educational setting.

TRANSFERENCE

Freud's (1912a, 1915) papers on transference represent the first definitive works in this area. Freud's own struggle to understand his work with his patient Dora (1905) drew attention to the process through which repressed longings anchored in unfulfilling past experience found expression in fantasy directed toward the therapist. The vitality of transference as a psychoanalytic construct has been emphasized by many subsequent authors, including Schwaber (1985), Stone (1984), and especially Gill (1982), whose extensive literature review and clinical work highlighted the centrality of transference to analytic treatment.

Because transference is conceived typically as the distortion of a contemporary relationship by the emergence of thoughts and feelings rooted in early developmental conflict, there needs to be some standard against which this distortion is assessed. It is here that conceptions of analytic neutrality become essential in establishing a base for evaluating the emergence of transference. What constitutes a neutral therapeutic stance, however, seems open to considerable debate.

Freud's technical papers (1912b, 1913, 1915) offered the standard guidelines for analytic neutrality. Langs (1982b), in his systematic approach to organizing clinical data, offered ground rules for establishing analytic neutrality that were similar to Freud's ideas. However, Langs also provided a strategy for evaluating breaks in neutrality that questioned the degree to which the client's unconscious perceptions of the therapist were grounded in fantasy rather than reality. Other psychoanalytic authors have also challenged the basic intrapsychic assumption of the classical model in which transference is conceived as a predominantly intrapsychic construct organized around unconscious fantasy constellations. Smith (1991), building on the rigorous standards of analytic listening set forth by Langs (1982b), also disagreed with Freud's construction of transference as grounded primarily in fantasy and distortion. In his work, Smith challenged Freud's seduction theory (Masson 1984), in which the idea of distortion was given precedence over reality as an organizing construct for experience. Smith takes the position that what are typically considered transference manifestations in much of the contemporary analytic literature are in fact

more accurately defined as reality-based, unconscious perceptions of the therapist's functioning. For both Langs and
Smith, deviations in analytic neutrality occur at much
greater frequency than usually thought.

Taking a middle-ground stance, Troise (1993) discussed
empirical findings that support the validity of transference
as a defensible psychoanalytic construct, but critiqued
Freud's idea that transference derived exclusively from
client reactions to analytic neutrality. Maroda (1994) questioned the sensibility of forced adherence to classical
neutrality. She critiqued the traditional idea of analytic
neutrality by arguing that rigid conceptions of neutrality
contribute to the therapist's inauthenticity. Instead she
argued that the authoritarian therapeutic stance by which
analytic neutrality has been defined historically "may
actually *distort and inhibit* the transference that would
have developed in a more reciprocal relationship" (p. 14,
italics original). According to Maroda, the very neutrality
that is meant to stimulate transference distortion may
itself be so distorting as to skew the transference. In sum,
the literature appears to have tied conceptions of transference to conceptions of neutrality, with different ways of
viewing transference and neutrality operable within the
context of analytically oriented treatments.

Classroom Applications

Several questions emerge when considering the application of transference to the classroom setting. First, is
transference a viable concept for the classroom? Second,
what is the standard of neutrality that can be used to gauge
the presence of transference manifestations? Third, how
can transference manifestations be identified by the classroom teacher? The first two questions can be answered
together; the third question requires a separate response.

Transference Viability and Teacher Neutrality

The viability of transference as a construct germane to the educational setting has been noted by many authors, including Basch (1989), Anna Freud (1935/1979), Harris (1966), and Zabarenko and Zabarenko (1974). It may be argued, for example, that the degree to which a student has an atypical reaction to a particular class with a particular teacher at a particular point in time may in part be the result of unconscious, parental introjects that have become attached to the teacher rather than a reaction to any salient behavior by the teacher—indulgence, deprivation, reprimand, or isolation—that would warrant the student's response. These responses would then be considered transference reactions in a relatively distinguishable sense.

The identification of transference manifestations, however, mandates a relatively clear conception of boundaries or frames that serve as the reality base against which transference can then be identified. In Chapter 4, I suggested a general framework for the classroom setting. The dimensions of the classroom framework help the teacher shape a style of relating to students that facilitates knowledge acquisition because of its benignly neutral tenor characterized by a prepared, informed, ethical, and respectful stance.

Even with these general guidelines for the classroom framework, it may be difficult to assess the state of this frame at any given point in time. Such difficulty is likely to exist because, unlike psychotherapy clients in analytic treatment, the structure of the traditional academic classroom does not lend itself to manifest representation of frame breaks by students. Instead the teacher usually enters the classroom, engages in some small talk with students, and then moves into the delivery of prepared material.

Under such conditions, the teacher is likely to operate

strictly within the vacuum of the classroom, remaining focused on teaching, and giving minimal, if any, consideration to the state of the classroom frame. Because most teachers characteristically hold conscious views of themselves as dedicated, caring, informed, and concerned with the welfare of their students, extreme reactions to a teacher are most likely to be perceived as transference based rather than emanating from a perceived lack of neutrality anchored in a break in the classroom frame. But because I also believe that the state of the classroom frame is susceptible to modification in a way that escapes the teacher's attention (e.g., a teacher's not being mindful of the possibility that having attended a party at a student's house may account for that student's subsequent anxiety in the teacher's presence), I offer the notion of ascribing *pure transference* reactions to students with this caveat to the teacher.

Transference Indications in the Classroom

If, however, the framework of the classroom is usually stable, how may the teacher identify student transferences? Identification of student transferences may proceed first by general categorization and second by delineation of exemplars within each category. Gill (1982), in his review of Freud's writings on transference, discussed two types of transference: a positive, facilitative transference and a transference that was tied to resistance. Both kinds of transference lend themselves to inferences about classroom transference.

First, in their positive form, student transferences may manifest in attitudes toward the teacher that are cooperative, engaging, and respectful of role. Students hand in work on time, come to class prepared, ask informed questions, and respect the teacher's professional role and boundaries. When positive transferences predominate, learning is fun, stress is manageable, and the teacher is seen as a basically benign person who helps students move through new content in a way that permits synthesis, insight, and professional development.

It is through an understanding of the second type of transference that indications of transference as resistance to learning take form. Resistances to learning that may be related to transference reactions to the teacher can be inferred through a variety of behavioral markers. Five reactions offer a representative sampling of the types of behaviors that can alert the teacher to the possibility of student transference. These behaviors include (1) frequent absence from class, tardiness, or both; (2) late submitting of assignments; (3) inappropriate exchanges; (4) requests for extrainstructional contact; and (5) failure to communicate directly.

Frequent Absence from Class, Tardiness, or Both

Students who miss class regularly or who always arrive well after class has begun may be indicating, through their absent or tardy behavior, transferential dynamics. Any number of acceptable reasons for a student's absence, including illness and family emergency, may be outside the scope of transference enactments in the classroom. Apart from these special circumstances, however, unconscious transference reactions to the teacher may influence decisions to miss class. For example, the failure to properly manage time that may lead a student to miss one teacher's class in order to put in extra time on work that is due for another course may actually speak to transference reactions on both fronts—poor time management around one teacher's requirements and the decision to miss another teacher's class. If this type of pattern is characteristic of a student, then transference issues become a plausible explanation for the absences. Similarly, chronic lateness not due to emergency also speaks to the possibility of transference as an underlying dynamic.

Late Submitting of Assignments

Students who frequently request extensions on assignments can also be understood in terms of transference reactions to the teacher. The specific content behind the transference process may be difficult to identify, but the recurrent theme of not being able to bring work to closure would appear to speak thematically to a conflict, quite possibly with passive-aggressive implications, around producing work within time constraints. Students who are late with assignments for reasons that are not the result of unexpected personal emergencies place demands on the teacher that extend the boundary of the classroom. In these cases, the teacher first must decide whether to grant the extension. Failure to do so may be interpreted by the student as being unusually rigid. The teacher's quick agreement to an extension, however, may send the student the message that different rules apply for different people. If the delay is granted, the teacher must then grade the student's work out of context. Grading work out of context means that the teacher may have to revisit evaluation criteria that were laid to rest a few weeks earlier. There is also the absence of other students' test answers to use for a comparative base around hairsplitting grading discriminations, as well as the possibility that the teacher may experience ambivalence about having to grade during a point in the semester at which he or she had anticipated a respite. By granting an extension of due date, the teacher may also be forced to grapple with questions about imposing a penalty on the late work and with fantasies about how the student will interpret the loss of points due to lateness. Ideally, the course syllabus specifies such parameters around deadlines and consequences. Even then, the student who presents work after deadlines have come and gone arouses certain thoughts and feelings in the teacher that may speak, on a deeper level, to an underlying transference dynamic related to the student's need for special considerations.

Inappropriate Exchanges

Students who, without seeming provocation, react inappropriately toward the teacher may be reacting in this manner because of transference stirrings. The types of reactions to which I am referring go beyond the strong but reasonable challenges to the teacher's position that actually characterize mature interplay between adult student and teacher. In the latter case, teacher and student may disagree, but there is an ability to process the interaction in a way that lends itself to a mutual understanding of the interpersonal sensitivities that get stirred periodically in the service of intellectual and personal growth. In some cases, however, there may be great difficulty in relating to the teacher. In the absence of any strong teacher stimulus for this behavior, it seems appropriately anchored within the realm of student transference. The range of such student reactivity includes, but is not limited to, sexualized and aggressive displays. These types of reactions to the teacher can rouse stress to uncomfortable levels, even when the teacher has access to concepts and consultants that help to mediate the intensity of the exchange.

Requests for Extrainstructional Contact

By extrainstructional contact, I refer to requests for contact with the teacher outside the scope of a defined learning context. Periodic tutoring requests that fall within office hours, phone contacts during work hours, class trips, and eating lunch with a student at a professional conference all represent appropriate contact with a teacher outside the class. These contacts are all in the service of the student's professional development and do not represent transference reactions in any extreme way. However, social invitations unrelated to classroom learning or requests to meet the teacher off campus for tutoring may each be reflective of an underlying transference dynamic in which the student seeks special attention from the teacher in a way that attempts to move the relationship beyond the realm of the classroom. Such requests pose a special concern to teachers who wish to remain supportive and fear being perceived as distant. A teacher can find rationalizations to support each behavior. From a psychoanalytic perspective, however, contact with students outside the parameters of a defined learning situation may result in the accentuation of the student's transference reaction to the teacher in such a way that new expectancies then emerge with the anticipation that they, too, will be gratified.

Failure to Communicate Directly

There are times during a student's experience in a program that he or she may seek the consultation of an academic adviser in order to deal with an awkward interpersonal situation that has arisen either with another student or with a teacher. In these situations, the adviser serves as a trusted professional in a mentoring context whose role it is to provide the student with some general counsel on how to handle a novel situation that may be compromising the learning experience of an advisee.

A student's need to seek the counsel of a faculty adviser during a period of crisis related to academic performance is different, however, from the decision to communicate to a teacher through another student. Students who tend to do their talking to the teacher through other students, friends, or family members may be doing so because of transference fantasies associated with direct teacher contact. For instance, a student who is absent from class and has another student (or a spouse) call on his or her behalf ("Tell him that I'm home sick") or who requests that another student be a spokesperson for conveying course concerns to the teacher ("When you see her, tell her that I'm uncomfortable with . . .") presents as being reluctant to engage the teacher directly. Not only does such indirect communicating bode poorly for establishing and maintaining relationships with teachers, but it sets the stage for serious miscommunication. Students who have other students talk for them or otherwise serve as their conduits with teachers inevitably *do* have contact with the teacher. This contact occurs when the teacher thinks about them in isolation from other students precisely because of their reluctance to represent themselves directly. By refraining from direct contact they stir the teacher's curiosity and lead to speculations about transference dynamics that may underlie the seemingly avoidant behavior.

Transference Interventions

For the most part, opportunities to intervene around inferred transference dynamics in the traditional classroom setting are few and far between. Situations that would be ripe for a transference intervention are uncommon because of the design of the academic setting. In order for there to be such an intervention, there would need to be privacy, a rapport with the student, and sufficient clinical material to warrant an interpretation from which the student would actually be able to benefit. Thus, the teacher may instead have to subject the wish to intervene to self-analysis and come up with another strategy for managing the tempting urge and its underlying dynamics. Should, however, a situation arise that lends itself to an interpretation of transference, the results can be extremely valuable both to student and teacher.

A student requested an appointment with a teacher prior to an examination in order to better understand certain lecture material. Despite the teacher's prolonged and patient review of seemingly straightforward didactic content that clearly was within the student's grasp, the student became openly distressed and voiced annoyance at the teacher. Discussion of the student's reaction led the student to spontaneously disclose that personal issues tied to a fear of failure rooted in the student's relationship with a parent had been clouding the student's receptiveness to the teacher's effort to help. The student had associated father with teacher and was quite anxious about not succeeding on the test. The teacher helped the student process this reaction. Subsequently, the student performed quite well on the examination, including the part of the examination that dealt with the content area in which the student had sought tutoring.

This example helps to illustrate the way a teacher's sensitive handling of a transference reaction can reduce the student's stress level and permit a meaningful integration of content that the student had initially experienced as being difficult to understand. The fact that the student performed well on the test may be taken as a further index of the way the reduction in conflict tied to the teacher permitted greater use of the cognitive and affective resources involved in answering the examination questions. The example also illustrates that conflict rooted in the past can become attached to the teacher in a way that compromises the student's learning.

COUNTERTRANSFERENCE

Within the psychoanalytic lexicon, few terms have as much vitality as *countertransference*. In a general sense, countertransference has been classically defined as the therapist's reactions to the client that are non-neutral. Challenges to this traditional conception of countertransference notwithstanding, the great appeal of countertransference to all psychoanalytic therapists would appear to rest with its defining quality as a source of clinical data; that is, countertransference reactions help the therapist define critical moments in the therapeutic relationship.

Despite its universal draw in analytically oriented work, countertransference eludes definitive conceptions. Questions about how to define neutrality, how to work clinically with the content of countertransference reactions, and the extent to which such reactions inform the therapy process have all been the subject of an extensive literature debate that has captured both the appeal of and the confusion surrounding countertransference as a clinical phenomenon (Langs 1976a,b, Maroda 1994, Smith 1991, and Tansey and Burke 1989).

Emerging from this literature are several key, interrelated issues that appear to polarize along temporal and spatial lines the substantive concerns pertaining to countertransference in clinical work. For example, are countertransference manifestations omnipresent or neurotic? Can they be identified as both realistic and distorted at different points in time? Should they be teased out, or are they potentially beneficial? Should they be kept private or disclosed? Should they be processed systematically or discerned through individualistic self-analytic strategies? Do they exist both situationally and in more enduring forms? Are their most salient characteristics manifested to the client through direct interaction with the therapist or through the therapist's management of the structural aspects of the therapeutic setting? Is their impact on the client best inferred by examining clinical material of which the client is conscious (i.e., the client's direct statements to the therapist), clinical material of which the therapist is conscious (the therapist's recognition of the arousal of angry, sexual, or depressed feelings toward the client), or unconscious narrative (the client's disguised allusions to the therapist through displaced derivatives)?

Answers to these questions shape not only the therapist's approach to clients, but to the entire therapeutic transaction. How the therapist thinks, feels, and reacts at any moment in time is colored by the way he or she answers questions about the nature of countertransference. With this degree of potency, countertransference has clearly earned its niche as a hall-of-fame construct within the arena of psychoanalytic theory and treatment.

Classroom Applications

An additional question that arises from a review of the countertransference literature is the relevance of countertransference in the teaching situation. Is countertransference a useful concept for the psychoanalytically oriented teacher? To this, I answer yes. Countertransference does indeed inform the teacher's work with students. What, then, are the implications of countertransference for classroom teaching and learning?

Countertransference Viability and Teacher Neutrality

The teacher's countertransference can be understood as a form of psychological resistance that impedes classroom learning. In this definition, there is a parallel to the notion of negative student transference as also representing a type of resistance to learning. Further, if the stability of the classroom framework represents a type of reality against which transference reactions can be assessed, then breaks in this same framework are the clearest gauge for evaluating modifications in the teacher's neutrality and for identifying countertransference. Thus, for purposes of discussion, the teacher's countertransferences are those thoughts, feelings, and actions that impede student learning and that are most powerfully manifested through breaks in the teaching hold, or framework.

Clearly there are hypothetical parallels that exist in the authority lines drawn between the teacher's relationship to administrative authority and the teacher's authority in the classroom with students. In this regard, there may be instances in which the teacher plays out with students elements of conflictual identification stirred through limitations in the holding environment within the educational setting. For example, a teacher whose phone remains broken despite several work orders submitted to an administrator may unconsciously enact an identification with the slow-to-act administrator by taking excessive time to return examinations to a group of students. These types of enactments, addressed in a general way in Chapter 3, represent the powerful, systemic communications that resonate throughout an institutional setting.

Because countertransference as a construct is applied to the role of authority in any clinical relationship and because teaching embodies elements of a clinical relationship, however, the teacher's countertransference can be best understood in relation to students.

Countertransference Indications in the Classroom

In keeping with the previous discussion of the stable classroom framework as a boundary for the identification of the transference reactions in students, I have identified a sampling of breaks in the classroom framework that teachers may be able to recognize from their own experiences. These breaks can be taken as manifestations of countertransference. Some such examples have already been provided in Chapter 4 as part of a general presentation of the organization of the teaching framework in the traditional classroom setting. The very same student behaviors that can be ascribed to transference dynamics can also be identified as countertransference dynamics in teachers, depending upon the state of the teaching framework and the teacher's sensitivity to it.

Frequent Absence from Class, Tardiness, or Both

Because the teacher's responsibility to students requires his or her presence in class, frequent absences and tardiness may be presumptive of a countertransference reaction. To be sure, there are occasions when the teacher is either late for, or misses, an occasional class due to illness, emergency, or competing professional obligations, including attending conferences or being delayed in leaving a meeting prior to the start of class. Although students are usually accepting of these behaviors without much conscious fanfare, they still resonate with the unconscious implication of countertransference enactments by the teacher. For instance, the 20-minute rule, which many classes seem to adopt in the spirit of a vacation day, frees students to leave the class if the teacher has not arrived within 20 minutes after the designated starting time. On the surface, there may be excitement, confusion, or annoyance surrounding the possible absence. There is also the thought of not being held accountable when the teacher is delayed beyond this time frame. On a deeper level, however, the 20-minute rule speaks to a fight-fire-with-fire approach in which students express anger over feeling abandoned by the teacher by themselves abandoning the classroom and, symbolically, the teacher.

Such implication is magnified should absence or tardiness become a routine way in which the teacher fulfills classroom obligations to students. The teacher who misses several classes, or who is routinely late for class, conveys several messages to students about his or her concern for the welfare of students. Included among the possible implications embedded in chronic lateness or poor attendance are teacher apathy, depression, and anxiety associated with student contact. The teacher who is aware of any frame breaks along these lines may, for example, be able to understand a particular student's subsequent lateness not as transference per se, but as a reaction to the teacher's lateness and management of the frame in this regard. In contrast, the teacher who does not attend to the impact of countertransference dynamics may instead feel slighted or angered by this same student's lateness and attribute transference issues to the student.

Lack of Preparation

Ideally, the teacher comes to each class prepared to teach. Although each class is different from the previous class, some general principles govern adequate preparation. Adequate teacher preparation for class may include reading the same material that students have been assigned to read and developing an orderly lesson plan that matches syllabus content. A well-prepared teacher also has sufficient breadth and depth of content within the discipline to respond in an informed manner to the range of questions that can arise during the class. Inadequate preparation is therefore reflected by omission in any of these areas and is suggestive of an underlying countertransference response. Implications of this type of countertransference include difficulty managing anxiety associated with course material in the context of having to present this material to a group of students.

Few things hinder student learning more than a teacher who presents lecture material in a confusing manner or who seems insufficiently informed about the topic under review. Confusing lectures breed confusing lecture notes.

Teachers who seem unfocused, who engage in frequent digressions from lecture material without alerting students, or who read directly from texts without leaving much room for either eye contact or dialogue can leave students feeling perplexed. How are they to identify essential information if distanced by the paucity of exchange and uncomfortable about asking the teacher for help? Teachers who react defensively when asked questions can make students feel anxious about voicing opinions in class.

The absence of adequate class preparation by the teacher impacts students differently. Such impact may be evidenced through the exaggeration of typical character trends in students that emerge when expected supplies are withdrawn. Some students overcompensate and work on their own, whereas others become mired in uncertainty and react dependently by seeking direction from classmates. In both cases, the teacher's countertransference has the effect of making students feel distanced as learners.

Inappropriate Exchanges

One aspect of a secure teaching frame involves respectful dialogue with students. Respectful dialogue involves attentive listening, thoughtful replies, sensitivity to ethical issues when interacting with students, and the presentation of instructive feedback in a way that facilitates learning. Breaks in this aspect of the teaching framework would appear to signal, at the very least, the teacher's difficulty with affect regulation and an insensitivity to the professional boundaries that define teacher and student.

In addition, fractious or otherwise inappropriate exchanges with students may occur along with other breaks in the teaching frame. For instance, situations in which the teacher and student strongly disagree over the grading consequences for verbal participation in class can lead to uncomfortable encounters for all involved. In this situation, the teacher may have implicit expectations about participation, but has neither articulated this expectation in the syllabus nor developed reasonable criteria for distinguishing quality of participation. Because some students tend to speak up in class more than other students, there may be a temptation to keep track of quality of participation impressionistically. Thus, those students who ask questions are perceived as the most active participants, while those students who remain relatively silent are perceived as less involved. In reality, students who tend toward little verbal involvement in class may do so for any number of reasons, including shyness, preference for silent deliberation versus active or anxious questioning, or sufficient grasp of the course material that precludes the necessity of initiating dialogue in class. As such, quiet students may be equally engaged by the material, but display this involvement differently.

In the event that such a student is, however, graded down because of the perception of limited participation, questions can emerge that pose direct challenge to the teacher's sense of fair play. Examples of the types of questions that students may raise in response to a perceived lack of clarity concerning participation include: "What are you defining as criteria for full credit for participation?" "How is this measured?" "How can upwards of 20 percent of a course grade be allotted to student participation under these ill-defined circumstances?"

In sum, students may pose strong challenges to the teacher's integrity in situations where punitive consequences are administered in the seeming absence of forewarning. In response to these challenges, the teacher may confront the students' reactions in strong terms and react defensively. Strong tone and defensive reactions by the teacher can leave students feeling powerless, dismissed, exasperated, embittered, and mistreated. If, on the other hand, the teacher is able to hear the student out with an openminded sensitivity to a possible break in the teaching frame as a trigger for the student's complaint, then the opportunity to learn from, and provide a model of conflict resolution to, the student is enhanced greatly.

Requests for Extrainstructional Contact

Ideally, teachers limit their contact with students to the classroom, office hours, and other educational contacts and professional activities that serve to foster the students' learning and professional development. With these markers serving as a boundary and buffer for student–teacher contact, countertransference can be inferred as being present in teachers who press for contact with students outside of this defined learning context. For instance, a teacher who seeks to develop student relationships that have no immediate referent to the student's educational pursuits may do so with the rationalization that such relationships are part of student socialization.

Efforts to establish social or professional relationships with students, however, leave the teacher vulnerable to reduced objectivity and perceived abuse of power. One example of the type of relationship that creates these vulnerabilities involves efforts to engage students socially, such as through the subtle solicitation of invitations to student parties. Similar efforts to seek the students' involvement in a nonteaching professional relationship may be suggested by the teacher's passing out professional business cards at the beginning of a class rather than just putting a phone number in the syllabus. These and similar occurrences that take the teacher beyond the scope of the students' academic learning can precipitate serious problems and consequences for the student–teacher relationship. With an eye on the implications of keeping the teaching framework relatively stable, the teacher may be able to check temptations to alter relationships with students in the service of fostering student trust and protection within the classroom setting.

Failure to Communicate Directly

Within the context of a stable teaching framework, teachers work to communicate directly with their students. Direct communication involves trying to achieve uniform instruction, processing student concerns through appropriate listening and responding, taking responsibility for all grading decisions, and, in a broader sense, attempting to minimize miscommunication about course material and requirements. Examples of indirect communication include asking one student to convey the teacher's concerns about another student to that second student (also a break in confidentiality), rerouting student concerns to administrators prematurely without first making an effort to resolve these concerns directly, permitting assistants to grade examinations or papers without first having cleared grading criteria with the teacher, and keeping irregular office hours that leave students calling clerical staff in order to locate the teacher during time of need.

Indirect communications to students signal countertransference and render the teacher susceptible to being perceived as elusive, enigmatic, vague, and uneasy with authority. Defensively, the teacher may react to these impressions by identifying students as being needy, overly sensitive, or difficult. Such defensiveness helps the teacher manage anxiety attendant to direct communication, but does not represent a particularly adaptive response to student complaints. In contrast, efforts to communicate directly with students convey the teacher's openness, accessibility, and willingness to work toward a stable learning environment.

Frame Interventions

Langs (1985) has described and illustrated the positive effect of holding the therapy frame stable even when clients pressure the therapist to modify the boundaries of the relationship. Similarly, the teacher may also be pressured occasionally by students to change the nature of the teaching framework. Examples of how students may press the teacher for a modification in the teaching framework include requests to either cancel class or end class early, reduce reading requirements, and make individual exceptions that disturb the neutrality of the teaching frame. When such requests are made in response to a relatively secure frame, they most likely reflect student anxiety associated with the security of a stable hold.

A student received a course grade that precluded tuition reimbursement by the student's employer. The student asked to meet with the teacher to discuss the grade. A brief discussion ensued during which the teacher delineated grading criteria and offered a convincing rationale for the student's grade. The student acknowledged the appropriateness of the grade, but continued to exert pressure on the teacher to modify it so that the tuition support might be secured.

The teacher wavered openly but refused to change the grade. Preoccupied with the student's financial problems for several days after the meeting and thinking about revising the decision, the teacher sought professional consultation to determine whether the decision to hold steadfast to grading criteria was indeed the appropriate action. The consultation led the teacher to consider the possibility that the distress felt over hurting the student's chance for reimbursement was a reaction-formation against anger over having been challenged by the student. The teacher had been challenged vigorously, felt angry, and defended against this anger introjectively through self-blame. Another, less obvious, source of anger was the teacher's reaction to the student's financial dependence despite being able to afford tuition independent of reimbursement. The student had commented that personal income was available to pay for the course, though getting reimbursement would obviously be preferred.

The teacher also became aware of the underlying shame that the student probably felt in response to receiving a grade that did not meet employer standards. Although the student had not voiced this concern during the discussion, it became apparent to the teacher that there was meaning attached to the grade that had consequence for the student's self-esteem. The student's grade would have to be forwarded to the employer, who would see the grade and then decline reimbursement.

The consultation had the positive effect of deepening the teacher's sensitivity to the various issues that were associated with the reaction to the student's request for a grade change. To change a grade under these circumstances, however, would be an obvious violation of grading policy. Based upon the information gleaned through the consultation, the teacher was able to place the student's request for a grade change into a more mature perspective and decided to let the grade stand in keeping with the established grading policy.

In this example, the teacher's use of professional consultation helped to integrate dynamics underlying the teacher's conscious struggle around the grading decision. Modification of the grade in response to pressure from the student would have represented a collusion with the student's seeming sense of fiscal entitlement as well as a reaction to the underlying shame associated with the low grade. The teacher's integrity would have been wide open for critique if and when other students became aware of the decision. Moreover, the example illustrates the challenges of containing and processing the strong affects aroused in connection with student requests for special considerations related to grading. Such requests are usually presented with an appeal to the teacher's sensitivity to exceptional circumstances and can touch the teacher in a very personal way. The teacher's readiness to oblige such requests on demand would clearly extend beyond the scope of good teaching practice. Uniform dismissals, on the other hand, without deliberating on the uniqueness of each situation, would deny the teacher opportunities to appreciate the breadth of issues with which students struggle amid a competitive academic environment.

PROJECTIVE IDENTIFICATION

Projective identification is yet another crucial psychoanalytic construct whose interpersonal implications have been discussed extensively in the literature. In general, projective identification is an interactional process between subject and object in which subject projects into object, identifies with the projected content, and then re-introjects in modified form the original projected content. Similar to the literature on countertransference, however, that on projective identification has inspired various conceptions. Included are conceptions of projective identification as (1) a mode of discharge for tensions associated with fantasy constellations—an object relational approach (Crisp 1986, Grotstein 1986, Ogden 1979); (2) a selfobject function located within a self psychology–object relational paradigm (Adler and Rhine 1988); (3) a primitive defensive mechanism with adaptive aspects operating along psychotic, borderline, and neurotic levels of personality organization (Kernberg 1987); and (4) a normal mode of communication with defensive and adaptive properties that can be systematically analyzed through a stage-processing model (Tansey and Burke 1989, Yalof 1991).

Projective identification may thus be described as an interpersonal strategy such that it (1) involves communication between subject and object in which subject uses object to help organize and then recover in more adaptive form conflictual psychic content; (2) is applicable across broad diagnostic groups and theoretical camps; (3) operates outside conscious awareness; (4) embodies elements of fantasy and reality; (5) overlaps the intrapsychic maneuver of projection proper; (6) can be analyzed through either systematic or personalized self-analytic strategies; and (7) serves both adaptive and defensive ends.

Classroom Applications

As an interpersonal process, projective identification can also be understood as the vehicle for the communication of transference and countertransference content, with implications for the relationship between student and teacher. As such, the same types of identificatory experiences and dyadic patterns that operate within psychotherapy can be applied to the selective classroom interactions between teacher and student.

The two central types of identification that operate in the projective identification cycle are *concordant* (subject and object experience similar affect states) and *complementary* (subject and object hold different psychological states). In their work on projective identification, Tansey and Burke (1989) have reviewed the historical roots of these two types of interpersonal identifications in the context of three dyadic object relational patterns of victim and victimizer. First, in the concordant victim–victim dyads, the client is identified with the role of victim in relation to a sadistic internal object representation and projects this victim identification into the therapist, who then identifies with the victim role. In this situation, the client may, for example, feel depressed, and the therapist begins to notice the onset of depressive feelings within himself or herself.

Second, in the complementary victimizer–victim pattern, the client is identified with the sadistic internal object and projects into the therapist the conflictual self-representation of victim. In this second situation, the client may, for example, berate the therapist, who recoils in response to the client's aggression. Third, in another complementary victim–victimizer pattern, the client is identified with the self-representation of victim, and the therapist takes on the sadistic object representation of victimizer. Here the therapist may begin to get angry with the client much in the same way that the client had experienced the victimizing internal object representation. In each of these three instances there are opportunities for the therapist to process and work clinically with projective identifications in a way that illuminates underlying client dynamics emerging in the treatment (Tansey and Burke 1989).

An example of applying different identifications and dyadic patterns of self-representation and object representation in the classroom occurs in a situation of a student whose continual yawning in class annoys the teacher, who reacts by avoiding the student's gaze. The student's yawning is just one manifestation of the distancing types of nonverbal behaviors that the student has manifested throughout the course. Because the yawning is noticeable and detracts from the teacher's usual sense of buoyancy, the teacher begins to perceive the student as being difficult to reach and feels annoyed. In conjunction with feeling annoyed, the teacher has the retaliatory fantasy of unexpectedly calling on the student for input, but refrains from this action. (Here the teacher is struggling with the fantasy of retaliating angrily in response to growing discomfort with a complementary identification of the victimizer–victim variety. In this identification, the teacher perceives the student as a victimizer who has made the teacher feel victimized through the distancing behaviors.)

Upon further deliberation about the events transpiring with the student, the teacher examines the state of the teaching frame and identifies it as being relatively stable. That is, the teacher is unable to identify any specific break in the frame that may be impacting the student in a way that can explain the type of interaction unfolding in the classroom. The teacher has been appropriately responsive to the few comments that the student has made during the course, despite the mildly irritating quality of the student's regular nonverbal displays of lethargy. Other aspects of the teaching frame seem to be intact.

As part of this line of inference, the teacher next considers the possibility that transference dynamics, triggered by the relatively stable frame of the class and manifested through a nonverbal projective identification, may be connected to the student's behavior and its disquieting impact on the teacher. In processing this reaction, the teacher speculates about the possibility that the student's yawning reflects an unconscious effort to distance the teacher. Yet the student has caused the teacher to take notice by virtue of the impact on the teacher of the nonverbal gesturing.

Because the teacher does not know anything about the student's personal history that would illuminate the inference about transference dynamics, the interpretation is kept general and focused on the distancing aspect of the teacher's immediate experience with the student. Here the teacher speculates that the exchange with the student may represent a possible reenactment of an earlier pattern in the student's life in which the student felt distanced by a parent at points when the student was trying to make an important point. This particular speculation appeared to fit the teacher's experience of feeling distanced by the student in a manner that was consistent with a victimizer–victim object-relational paradigm.

Continuing along these lines, the teacher speculates further about the interactional dynamics behind the student's yawning. In this regard, the defensive aspect distances the teacher, whereas the adaptive aspect of the student's yawning, by creating an air of apathy, may be protecting the student against active involvement with the teacher. The teacher is also aware, however, of having become somewhat preoccupied with the student. At this point, the teacher tentatively concludes that while the student has sought to distance the teacher as a way of minimizing involvement, there may also be an underlying desire for contact with the teacher of which the student is unaware.

The teacher uses this formulation as a way of gaining a deeper appreciation of the student's behavior. Options for dealing with the student include approaching the student after class and sharing observations of the student's behavior as a way of opening up communication or respecting the student's need to keep distance. Both alternatives breathe life into the student–teacher relationship and leave the teacher feeling less disturbed by the distancing aspects of the student's yawning. Here there is a movement toward a concordant identification that involves empathy with the student's need to manage psychological distance in relation to the teacher and away from the retaliatory fantasy that had begun to emerge earlier in the class period.

Had the teaching framework been broken and had the teacher been aware of such a break, then the above formulation would have taken on a different meaning. For instance, the student's reaction could be conceptualized in relation to the distancing aspects of the frame break itself and, by implication, of the teacher's countertransference. A reanalysis of the same material to which the aforementioned transference implication was ascribed would now suggest that the teacher was the victimizer and the student was the victim. An interpretation of this scenario may hold the teacher responsible for having precipitated a reality event—the frame break—that may have contributed to this student's distancing behavior. The student identified with the victim role and responded by behaving apathetically in class.

Systemic Applications of Projective Identification

Projective identification can also be used clinically to conceptualize systemic dynamics within an organizational structure (Shur 1994), for instance, by illustrating the processes through which administrators, teachers, and students receive and react to conflictual identifications and the ways this cycle of communication can ultimately serve to stabilize organizational dynamics.

In developing the annual academic calendar, a mistake was made by an administrator that escaped initial double check. Using the academic calendar to schedule classes, a teacher had planned an examination date that had to be rearranged when, subsequent to the distribution of the calendar, the administrator noted the error. The primary consequence of this error for students was that the examination had to be pushed one week ahead of the original schedule. The teacher reacted anxiously and tried to fit two lectures into one class. Students felt pressured but complied with the teacher's request to forge ahead with the material. Examination grades were lower than the teacher expected, with several bright students seeming confused in response to a question that the teacher thought well within their grasp.

After grades were returned, students voiced anger with the way the teacher had proceeded to forcefeed material without adequate time for synthesis. They felt that they had been victimized. The teacher, while hurt by their response, acknowledged that they had good reason to feel angry. Later that same day, the teacher voiced concern to the administrator who had prepared the calendar; this person, too, was remorseful and appreciative of the teacher's remarks. The administrator told the teacher that a new system of checks and balances was being developed to ensure that no such calendar oversights occurred down the road. The teacher felt positive about the administrator's response.

At the start of the next class, the teacher offered students a brief take-home test that gave them the opportunity to revisit material from the examination. The second examination due date was left to the discretion of students, provided that it was completed within a three-week period. Students were appreciative of this offer and understood it as the teacher's effort to right a situation that had gone awry.

In this example, the role of projective identification and the modification of the projected themes can be traced through the line of exchange between administrator, teacher, and student. First, the teacher enacted a victim position in relation to the victimizing administrator by not taking action on the scheduling conflict prior to the examination date. Second, the teacher identified with the victimizing role by forcing material on students, who felt victimized.

Things began to change, however, after the teacher returned the grades. In response to feeling victimized, students responded in strong voice about the teacher's having taken advantage of them because of the scheduling dilemma. Students worked maturely with their reaction to having been cast into the role of unwitting victim by stirring the teacher into the victim role. In turn, the teacher became sensitized to the way students felt about the examination process. Of equal importance was the teacher's increased sense of fortitude that came from this identification with student assertiveness. The teacher not only felt the brunt of the misdeed, but was able to present concerns to the administrator in a mature way that opened dialogue beyond the formal memorandum circulated after the calendar error was noticed. The teacher's decision to offer students a more benign examination forum would appear to reflect efforts to redress fracture in the teaching frame in response to a revised conception of the conflictual interactional pattern shaped by the projective identification process.

CHAPTER 7

Teaching Clinical Courses

The psychoanalytic educator who teaches clinical courses is invariably sensitized to student phenomenology. Clinical courses that address different facets of theory, technique, diagnosis, and application are relevant to the professional development of mental health students. These courses prepare students for the myriad of practice dilemmas and decisions that define clinical work.

Because of their relevance to practice, clinical courses represent the bread and butter of the academic curriculum. Insofar as they carry weight in identifying a student's preparedness to move beyond didactic and experiential training and into autonomous practice, performance in clinical courses is likely to influence a student's self-esteem. For example, a student's weak performance in a course that deals with theory and technique hits at the heart of an important competency. Although a certain amount of rationalization may help explain away a low grade, the meaning of the grade itself still resonates painfully on a deep level for students who envision themselves functioning as independent clinical practitioners. In contrast, practitioner-oriented students may be able to rationalize weak performance more easily in a statistics course by claiming, albeit not necessarily accurately, that the course does not have immediate relevance to hands-on clinical work.

It is the responsibility of the teacher to help students see clinical relevance in any given course. In order to appreciate the meaning that a particular course has to students, the teacher of clinical courses strives to empathize with the nuance of student experience. Such empathic responding goes beyond what can be accessed through a review of course evaluations and seeks to locate meaning in the underlying themes that arise for teacher and student in different clinical courses.

Because such themes are inferred by the teacher from classroom observation and student comment, their identification involves the type of clinical skill that the psychoanalytically informed teacher brings to the class. Further, different courses make different demands on teacher and student. Consequently, the way a student experiences the course's content and the course teacher differs across the different content domains that comprise a curriculum in mental health. Nevertheless, an overriding question for the psychoanalytic educator who wants to understand the nature of student experience in different courses may be framed as follows: How are students experiencing my course?

Reviewing the clinical courses of Projective Personality Assessment, Abnormal Behavior, Psychoanalytic Theory and Therapy, and Clinical Seminar is a way of sampling underlying themes that speak to student phenomenology. Because these four courses are designed to assist students in learning about the unconscious experiences of clients, they also provide a foundation for learning about the unconscious experiences of student and teacher from a psychoanalytic perspective.

PROJECTIVE PERSONALITY ASSESSMENT

Projective personality assessment has strong ties to psychoanalytic theory. Projective tests, with their relatively ambiguous test stimuli, lend themselves to psychoanalytic exploration. In the absence of familiar stimulus cues, minimal task directions from the examiner, and no right or wrong answers, these tests encourage the client to impose structure on the test stimuli by projecting internal dynamics onto them. Examples of projective tests are the thematic apperception test (TAT) (Murray 1938), in which the client makes up stories to explain scenes on picture cards; the Rorschach test (Exner 1993), in which the client responds to a series of inkblots with minimal direction from the examiner; and various types of figure-drawing tests (Groth-Marnat 1990), in which the client is asked to draw pictures of self and others. In this regard, projective testing differs from the unambiguous test stimuli and clear response expectations that define objective tests. However, even such objective tests as the Wechsler intelligence scale (Rapaport et al. 1968) and the Bender visual–motor gestalt test (Groth-Marnat 1990, Koppitz 1975) reveal underlying dynamic themes that speak to a projective element.

Projective Testing in Clinical Training

The projective test format has some commonality with psychoanalytic therapy in that the therapist's relatively neutral stance stimulates the emergence of the client's inner world into the client–therapist relationship. Indeed, projective testing has a firm anchor in psychoanalytic theory. Beginning with the seminal works of Rapaport and colleagues (1968) and Schafer (1948, 1954), psychoanalytic theory has been applied to personality tests in order to give diagnostic findings theoretical direction. Developments in psychoanalytic theory in the areas of ego psychology, object relations, and self psychology have been reflected in the projective test literature (Allison et al. 1968, Berg 1984, Kissen 1986, Kwawer et al. 1980, Lerner 1991, Schafer 1967, Sugarman 1981).

Projective testing has appeal for different mental health training programs. For example, in clinical psychology, projective testing has been a staple in program curricula and is considered to be a highly valued skill by internship training directors (Tipton et al. 1991). Many counseling psychologists also value and use projective tests as part of their professional work (Fitzgerald and Osipow 1986). Even in subdoctoral counselor training programs, there is strong student interest in learning about projective tests (Watkins et al. 1990). The readiness of training programs to offer projective testing courses suggests their importance to a student's professional development.

Student Phenomenology in Projective Test Courses

One striking limitation in the projective test literature has been the amount of attention given to the experience of students who are learning to administer, score, interpret, and report on projective tests (Yalof 1993). Yet learning about tests that bypass typical defenses and introduce a level of clinical subjectivity into the interpretive process seems to be both appealing and threatening to students. The appeal lies in the opportunity to study unconscious processes and synthesize their workings into a cohesive narrative that depicts a psychological profile. The threat lies in the demands that such a task presents. Whether it be learning complicated scoring systems, taking risks by applying sophisticated interpretive strategies, or refining prose and style, the student draws on his or her experiential base to derive meaning from test data. Further, the novelty of learning projective testing touches student phenomenology in a unique but relatively unexplored way.

In this regard, the teacher of personality assessment may raise the following question: With what do students learning projective tests struggle? In response to this question, there are three issues: (1) the teacher as wisdom figure, (2) the issue of believability when learning about projective tests, and (3) the student's identification with the projective test client.

The Teacher as Wisdom Figure

Helping students gain confidence in the interpretation of personality tests is the ultimate goal of the teacher. Good interpretation subsumes an understanding of personality dynamics, an ability to use concepts flexibly, an ability to reduce theoretical terms to descriptive language, and an appreciation for how test findings ultimately play out in different treatment settings.

Because of the highly specific nature of the skills needed to teach projective tests, the teacher is likely to be perceived by students as having a degree of wisdom that may exaggerate his or her actual knowledge as a clinician. Unlike other courses in which students may silently envision themselves as capable of soon being on a par with the teacher, the student of projective testing may instead ask "Will I ever learn this stuff to the teacher's level?"

This tendency to inflate the teacher's actual clinical competence may be most evident at the start of a course, when discrepancies in interpretive skill between student and teacher are most obvious. Which students, if any, can see themselves on a par with a teacher who has a firm grasp of the fine distinctions in scoring Rorschach shading variables? Which ones can see themes running through what on the surface seems to be a series of disparate TAT stories or identify signs of trauma in a single figure drawing or cross-validate inferences with data from different tests as well as from the client–tester interaction?

Idealization of the teacher's perceived wisdom has its assets and liabilities. Clearly, it provides the teacher with some leverage in getting across key points. In reality, however, no teacher desires a group of spellbound students. Thus, the teacher must search for indications that students are becoming more comfortable with the inference process underlying projective testing. Some signs of greater levels of comfort and confidence in students include increased frequency of students' insightful comments and the teacher's ability to take for granted concepts that initially required careful explanation.

Ultimately, bridging the gap between ideal and real images of the teacher can be accomplished by being patient with students as they work their way through a new knowledge base. The teacher also can achieve this end by developing examinations that require integration of classroom learning and give students a good shot at success. This would seem to be a sensible way of engaging students and stimulating their desire to achieve or surpass the level of their teacher.

The Issue of Believability

The teacher of projective personality tests often finds himself or herself trying to convince students of the verity, or believability, of the tests themselves. Student skepticism is fueled by the gaps between client test response and the interpretation of the response. This gap is represented by the multiple levels of abstraction that separate concrete test answer from clinical inference. For example, inferring that a dark hole centered in a tree trunk on a drawing suggests an underlying trauma may appear to be an overly speculative interpretation, and one that is unacceptable at first glance to many students unfamiliar with the rationale underlying projective test analysis. Similarly, a client's Rorschach response of "a black bat on the verge of attacking something" does not naturally lead the novice to think of the interpretation "Hostile ideational content may manifest through intensive, interactional projections possibly arousing within another person a sense of being attacked."

These are the types of interpretations that excite teacher and student because they access the client's underlying dynamics and help give direction to the relationship between presenting problem and unconscious factors. Yet students may react to these interpretations by asking, "How did you get that?" Clinical wizardry notwithstanding, the teacher must demonstrate to students that they, too, can begin to work confidently with projective test data. Promoting group discussion can encourage students to bring their clinical skills to the task of interpretation.

Drawing comparisons between the inferential process in psychotherapy, where therapists often speculate about unconscious implications of manifest content, and the interpretive process in projective testing can help students see the important continuity of learning to make clinical formulations that thread different parts of their training program. The teacher can also share his or her own method of interpreting projective test data so that students can track the teacher's reasoning process. For instance, in clarifying his or her thinking behind the interpretation of the "black bat" response, the teacher may say that "black" represents dysphoric affect, movement involves seeing something in the blot that is not really part of the blot—and is akin to the projection of ideational content— and "the verge of attacking" speaks to the precipice of rage. Thus the response condenses critical psychological features that reveal the form and content of the projected material. This type of sharing helps make projective tests believable to students and also demystifies the teacher, who demonstrates how clinical reasoning, not magical powers, underlies the interpretive strategy.

The Student's Identification with the Projective Test Client

The novelty of learning projective testing and the anxiety associated with this new learning render the student vulnerable in the classroom in a way that differs from other courses. For instance, learning that responses to an inkblot or to a simple picture can unearth hidden dynamics makes students think about clients' vulnerability when exposed to projective test procedures. In fact, such thinking is an expected part of a course in personality assessment. Because students are sensitized to their clients, they empathize with client vulnerability and may identify with it. Identification with client vulnerability would be an understandable reaction for students who feel vulnerable in a different type of learning situation. Certainly it is a reaction that warrants consideration.

In searching for reasons behind this type of identification, three points stand out. First, both client and student experience an element of transparency in response to projective testing. For clients, it takes the shape of feeling that the tester can look beneath the surface of manifest responses and into the deeper, more secretive layers of the psyche. For students, the element of transparency involves the anxiety that the teacher, with his or her high level of skill, is making penetrating insights about their psychological functioning and bypassing their defenses in the process. In this context, the teacher may be perceived not only as teaching the students, but also as conducting a silent analysis of each student, much in the same way that he or she analyzes the projective test data. In reality, both students and teachers engage in private assessments of each other throughout this and other courses. However, because of the nature of a course in projective testing, the teacher's clinical acumen may be elevated in the fantasy life of students, making it feel—at least for some students—that the teacher is picking up on the finer points of their personality.

Second, there is anxiety associated with the loss of control in the relative absence of traditional supports. For clients, the test process itself offers few clues as to what they should see and few reality checks as to whether their perceptions are presenting them in a sane light. For students, it is not the test itself, but the novelty of the learning task and the difficulty in bringing existing skills to bear on the interpretive process that can stimulate a sense of dyscontrol over the didactic material (and the grade).

Third, there is a sense of passivity and even victimization that binds client and student. Whereas the client takes projective tests at the recommendation of a referral source, the student is taking the class at the request of the psychology department. Neither client nor student gets involved with the therapist or psychology department, respectively, because of a commitment to projective testing. At moments of frustration or anxiety, a sense of feeling victimized may reign because of the transparency and dyscontrol that students experience by virtue of their involvement with projective tests.

Some signs that students are struggling with these issues may be excessive doubting of the merit of projective testing, including quibbling about psychometric properties vis-à-vis nonprojective measures, disputing the diagnostic yield of projective tests compared to clinical interviews, and strongly minimizing the role of unconscious factors in psychological functioning. Such concerns are most likely to emerge during the earliest phase of a course, when students are acclimating to the various learning demands of projective testing. Through these maneuvers, students seek to avoid being identified with tests that they fantasize may not be particularly beneficial to clients. On another level, by seeking to protect clients, students may also be seeking to protect themselves from the transparency, dyscontrol, and victimization themes that color the learning process.

ABNORMAL BEHAVIOR

A course in abnormal behavior is a staple in the mental health education curriculum. The usual purpose of the course is to familiarize students with a range of diagnostic categories (*DSM-IV* 1994) and the types of behaviors manifested by clients who fit these categories. A course in abnormal behavior may also include information about treatment implications, though the vast range of client needs that distinguish many of the diagnostic groups makes it difficult to do justice to treatment implications within a single course on abnormal behavior.

Above and beyond content, a course in abnormal behavior encourages students to think about their own behavior in ways that can be somewhat distressing but potentially useful in gaining mastery over course concepts and insight into their own personality dynamics. For example, by teaching the concepts of character, symptom formation, defense, and trauma, the teacher shapes the main themes that help students organize the course content. It may be difficult, however, to listen to lectures and read material that addresses these areas without also evaluating oneself in relation to the material under study. Attention to the material presented by the teacher also engages the student on a very personal level. Thus, while the student is working to integrate the content of the lecture and readings into a gestalt of psychopathology, there may also be another level of synthesizing at work that addresses the student's own dynamics and history. Three descriptive themes that help to capture the student's experience of being in a class on abnormal psychology are (1) self-diagnosis; (2) the intrusion of disturbing imagery, and (3) mastery strivings.

Self-Diagnosis

It is well known that medical students, upon initial classroom exposure to the various illnesses that plague people, become very sensitive to their own health and self-diagnose a variety of maladies. Students in mental health training programs may or may not be different from medical students in this regard; if one were to harbor a guess, however, it might be that they are more similar than different. Self-diagnosis is indeed part of the life of a mental health student. The content of a course in abnormal psychology underscores this observation.

The content of the abnormal psychology course stirs the waters of self-diagnosis by making students think intensively about the types of traumatic incidents and psychological vulnerabilities that define the human condition. If placed on a psychological continuum, people may be able to identify within themselves attenuated versions of many of the clinical features that bear the stamp of a verifiable psychiatric condition. Degrees of anxiousness, self-esteem fluctuations, mood variations, compulsivity, and defensiveness are, for example, selectively intensified in different diagnoses but are common to all individuals.

For this reason, it seems quite understandable that students engage in silent diagnosis of self and others throughout the duration of the course. Weekly exposure in class to the types of clinical features that denote psychopathology, especially if couched in clinical illustration, encourages the student's empathy with individuals in need of professional assistance. Moreover, the types of diagnostic groups that are typically represented—people with personality disorders, victims of trauma, substance abusers, those with schizophrenia—and the rich, clinical descriptions that convey these people to students would appear to arouse the student's fantasies about self and others in a way that is very natural. Silent self-diagnostic questioning may take the form of "What's my diagnosis?" Asking this question, however, without thinking about the significant others in one's life who may have contributed to the need to even ask this type of question is almost impossible.

The Intrusion of Disturbing Imagery

Raising questions pertaining to self-diagnosis would appear to be a natural sequela of the abnormal psychology course; many people who pursue advanced training in mental health do so as a reaction to life experiences that have exposed them to different types of psychological hardship (Guy 1987). Such questions may operate as background noise in the context of listening to a lecture, taking notes, asking questions, writing a paper, and participating in discussion. They call forth, however, images of disturbing events in the student's life.

These events may include conflicts with parents, siblings, spouses, employers, and any others tied to disturbing events in the student's life. Some such imagery may have been either partially or fully repressed prior to the abnormal psychology course, but can become increasingly and uncomfortably accessible to the student as the course unfolds. As a result, images of an alcoholic parent, a substance-abusing sibling, a schizophrenic cousin, an ex-roommate who exhibited a disquieting level of personality disturbance, or a depressed spouse may float in and out of the student's conscious awareness with unexpected frequency. The unearthing of this imagery has the potential value of providing the student with new opportunities for higher levels of mastery over conflictual events within the context of the course itself.

Mastery Strivings

For those students who revisit conflictual events during a course in abnormal psychology, there are opportunities for self-reflective work within the protective structure of a classroom situation. New awareness, or old awarenesses that now have different slants, can be brought into personal therapy or processed during supervision in ways that make clinical work more meaningful. In addition, examinations and term papers give students room to integrate these awarenesses with new concepts. New understandings gleaned from course concepts assist students in maintaining sufficient emotional distance from conflictual material while affording them the room to work creatively with new insights.

For teachers there is the knowledge that, apart from teaching content, their lectures are evoking important questions in students. These questions help the student anchor life experience to clinical situations, facilitate recollection of disturbing incidents in the student's personal life, and encourage new opportunities for self-reflection and insightful application within the classroom setting. For both student and teacher, there is a heightened appreciation for viewing psychopathology along a continuum of disturbance from which no person is immune.

PSYCHOANALYTIC THEORY AND THERAPY

Teaching a course in psychoanalytic theory and therapy poses many of the same challenges to the teacher as do teaching courses in projective personality assessment or abnormal psychology. For example, the teacher who can lecture with seeming facility on the nuances of analytic theory or who can organize clinical material into rich inferences that touch the depth of the analytic relationship is likely to be held in high esteem by students, who may question whether they will ever reach the teacher's perceived level of competence. Students also display skepticism about the very same clinical material that seems so intriguing during lecture and discussion. Such skepticism may take the following forms: "Does everything really relate to the therapist?" "Who can sit silently for so long, and doesn't it turn the patient off?" Moreover, students who are uneasy with the potency of analytic material may also experience an identification with the patient's presumed vulnerability within the analytic model.

For the teacher of psychoanalytic theory and therapy, a few prominent themes distinguish the subject from projective personality testing. Included among themes that organize the course for student and teacher are (1) misguided impressions of analytic theory and therapy that some students bring to the course, (2) problems posed by analytic terminology, and (3) the relevance of the analytic model to everyday practice.

Misguided Impressions about Analytic Theory and Therapy

There are several erroneous impressions about analytic theory and therapy that most teachers must deal with as part of teaching an introductory required course to students. Included here are the notions that all ideational content is subject to an aggressive and unremitting analysis and the therapist is cold and aloof. These are probably among the very same misconceptions that the teacher and his or her classmates grappled with at an early phase of their training. One aspect of teaching about psychoanalytic theory and therapy usually involves some proselytizing by the impassioned teacher, especially one who has moved beyond initial misgivings. Such a teacher expends some energy trying to draw students closer to contemporary analytic thinking in a way that encourages their appreciation of the psychoanalytic model from the teacher's perspective. To accomplish this end without coming across defensively to students, the teacher must be mindful of impressions about the analytic model that some students bring to the course.

The Notion of Aggressive and Unremitting Analysis

The fantasy that the psychoanalytic therapist is constantly analyzing the client can represent a source of irritation for students and one form of resistance to embracing the psychoanalytic orientation. A therapist cast in this light is likely to be perceived as aggressive and unempathic rather than as humanistic and caring. In reality, many clinicians are quite sensitive to underlying dynamics and regularly seek to understand these dynamics in the context of their clinical work. For example, rational-emotive therapists (Ellis and Grieger 1977) are also interested in the client's irrationality, fantasies about self in relation to others, and phenomenological state, even if they work with this material in a way that differs dramatically from the psychoanalytically oriented psychotherapist.

What distinguishes the analytic therapist from therapists of different orientations is the emphasis on understanding the client's experience of the therapist. Thus, while it is true that the analytic therapist is invested in analyzing hidden psychological content, so, too, are other therapists; they just approach it from a different angle. Quite possibly it is the fantasy of the vulnerable client laid bare before the dispassionate analytic therapist that spikes student anxiety about the aggressive quality of the therapist's work. As such, there may be an understandable but somewhat misconstrued idea among some students that the psychoanalytic psychotherapist constantly reads unnecessarily deep meaning into clients' comments and is not really different in direction from Freud (1905) in his aggressive pursuit of hidden meaning in his work with Dora.

There is some truth to the aforementioned image of the analytic therapist. When teaching students about psychoanalytic theory and therapy, the teacher covers such areas as the deduction of unconscious motives from conscious commentary, interpretation of dream imagery, discussion of the implications of sexual and aggressive drives, and the subtleties of transference and countertransference. Each of these elements of the analytic model looks for meaning beneath defenses, an area of exploration and study that can create discomfort for client, student, and teacher because it threatens to disrupt an individual's conscious representation of self and others.

In this regard, teaching students to search for hidden meaning as the root of manifest problems can only stir fantasies about the psychoanalytic therapist as someone who obsessively analyzes everything. In actuality, and this can be pointed out to students in a thought-provoking way, probably everyone who has an interest in learning about psychotherapy has on at least one occasion been guilty of overanalyzing. The tendency to overanalyze may in fact be characterological for some people and a sure source of contention in all relationships, analytic or not, unless this tendency to scrutinize is mediated by a sensitive understanding of context.

By presenting the temptation to analyze from the perspective of everyday occurrence, the teacher can help shape an image of the psychoanalytic therapist as someone who does what many people do, but with specific training and with disciplined attention to context and consequence. Without such a primer, the notion of unremitting analysis can quickly take on aggressive connotation and serve to further distance students who arrive in class with exaggerated conceptions of the therapist's role. Only by offering students a humanistic view of the analytic therapist along with a sensible and empathic strategy for organizing the client's material can the teacher begin to reach those students who seem overly sensitized to the aggressive aspects of psychoanalytic psychotherapy.

The Notion of the Cold and Aloof Therapist

Related to the fantasy of aggressive and unremitting analysis is the notion of a cold and aloof therapist. The depiction of the psychoanalytic therapist as someone who is emotionally distant and unavailable is an underlying, unpleasant theme that is potentially disruptive to student learning. Save for those students who have either been exposed to an empathic, analytically informed therapist or supervisor or who know someone who has been, initial impressions of the psychoanalytic psychotherapist are not likely to include such terms as empathy, support, humanism, and benignancy. These terms are attractive to students and therapists alike, but are not necessarily tip-of-the-tongue terms to use for the analytic therapist.

The teacher has to paint a picture of the psychoanalytic therapist consistent with theoretical and technical approaches that define a psychoanalytic approach to clinical work while helping students imagine a therapist who meets the criteria of a nurturant and kind human being.

These conceptions of the psychoanalytic therapist need not be mutually exclusive. Indeed, a seasoned psychoanalytic therapist is empathic, supportive, humane, and benign. Good interpretations, for example, in addition to explaining client complaints in light of conscious and unconscious factors, touch gently upon the client's inner world and sensitively address limitations in the therapist's functioning in a highly empathic manner that meets standards of psychoanalytic validation (Langs 1985, Tansey and Burke 1989, Trawinski 1990). Such interpretations are useful because they provide sufficient support for existing client defenses so as not to foster premature regression while encouraging a relaxation of defenses in order to permit higher-level synthesis of heretofore disparate psychic content.

Interpretations addressing client–therapist dynamics that are well timed, thoughtful, sensible, and gently delivered also present the therapist in a very humane light and foster an introjective identification with a benign figure. Students with limited exposure to contemporary analytic literature are not likely to have had the opportunity to bridge their existing thoughts about the role and functions of the psychoanalytic psychotherapist with present-day thinking. Consequently, the image of the analytic therapist may for these students remain the antithesis of the compassionate, insightful, and gentle clinician that the teacher hopes to promote.

These points are not easy to sell, however; they need to be made during the class through clinical illustrations and discussion of case material. Providing readings that focus on countertransference, integrating into case analysis the impact of the therapist's countertransference on the client's subsequent associations, and giving students learning tasks that help them become comfortable with countertransference can help win over students who may have entered the class thinking that the analytic therapist functions as a rigid automaton.

Problems Posed by Analytic Terminology

One of the challenges of teaching psychoanalytic theory and therapy is helping students understand psychoanalytic terminology. One is hard pressed to find an entry-level psychoanalytic text written in simple terms, with clear examples that anchor abstract concepts to a descriptive reality in a way manageable for students within the short-term time frame of an academic semester.

The teacher who introduces students to a strategy for working with psychoanalytic material in therapy may find himself or herself drawing on models that are wonderfully rich (Gill 1982, Langs 1982b, Rowe and Mac Isaac 1989, Tansey and Burke 1989) but that require ongoing translation of terminology. Indeed, clinical terms that the teacher may take for granted can befuddle the student. Moreover, when forced to define terms for students, the teacher, too, may open the window on questions anchored in his or her own training—questions that have lain dormant but that now require responses. Bright students raise bright questions, which not only mandate that the teacher think fast on his or her feet, but also require the teacher to openly grapple with the same issues over which students are seeking some degree of mastery.

There are any number of questions that emerge in class to challenge the teacher to define terms for students. For example, students may ask about the meaning of the classical position on countertransference. They may wonder if the classical position on countertransference is an ideal that is not really attainable, given the complexity of clinical material and the interpersonal nature of relations. Subsequent discussion may develop a line of reasoning that points out the value of learning to first identify and then neutralize strong reactions to clients. The ways in which different models foster this process in the therapist may then be reviewed.

Another example of a conundrum of terminology may arise in response to the introduction through readings and lecture of the concept of *projective identification*. A question may arise as to what projective identification really means. The teacher may find himself or herself working overtime to produce a plausible response. Indeed, many of the same questions surrounding the concept of projective identification noted in Chapter 6 become real concerns for students during a course. Is it an intrapsychic and primarily defensive structure, or can it be construed as an interactional process having both defensive and adaptive features? If it is intrapsychic, then can it really be distinguished from projection proper? Does all projection in fantasy contain an element of pressure on the internalized object with concomitant modification in subject, or does there have to be a real change in the intrapsychic state of the subject brought about by genuinely felt interpersonal pressure in order for there to be true projective identification? Is there an overarching construct that places both projection proper and the interactionally based projective identification on a continuum in order to account for the different phenomenological states attendant to each concept? If not, does psychoanalytic theory need such a construct?

These are but a few of the questions that the classroom teacher may have to confront in an attempt to clarify both to self and students the abstruse nature of analytic terminology. In addition to these questions, students who read Freud for the first time may struggle to understand his writing style and may need much clarification from the teacher. Students who are exposed to Kohut's work may react similarly. In short, the teacher must work hard to bring clarity where ambiguity is bound to exist in order to demystify key terms and help students understand them in light of everyday practice.

Relevance to Everyday Practice

In the changing world of clinical practice, the teacher of psychoanalytic theory and therapy must deal with the application of the psychoanalytic model to the managed care scheme and to the various field sites associated with the clinical training experience. Both are areas that pose some real problems for the psychoanalytically informed teacher primarily because of their seeming discord with the open-ended nature of the psychoanalytic model.

Managed Care

Within psychoanalytic psychology, Shore (1994) and Shulman (1994) have raised concerns about the role of psychoanalytic therapy in the managed care paradigm in a way that appears to capture the essence of the tension and sentiment surrounding the meaning of this relationship to psychoanalytic practitioners. In general, the psychoanalytic practitioner represents an outlier among the various service providers within the network of managed care. Challenges to the long-term, open-ended, and confidential nature of psychoanalytic work include fixed visits, controlled fees, and external reviewers who judge quality of work and influence decisions about continuation of treatment. Although there always exists an option to seek an exclusively private clientele who pay fees for services— thereby bypassing managed care and allowing for a high level of therapist autonomy—many students graduate into a job market where involvement with managed care may be a necessity in order to secure a caseload with predictable and reasonable remuneration.

In managed care, demands for psychoanalytic services will not be a top priority. Instead, therapy that is brief, problem focused, goal oriented, and quantifiable is what appeals to the managed care administrator. With these preferences, it is difficult to locate a place for psychoanalytic psychotherapy in managed care. The gradual reduction of symptoms, the loosening of defenses, the development of a meaningful attachment between client and therapist, all of which help define the psychoanalytic model, do not seem particularly conducive to the managed care approach.

For many students, the psychoanalytic model may have great appeal to their intuitive appreciation for the complexity of the human condition, but may not have equal appeal in encouraging short-term applications sensitive to the process-oriented and gentle manner that characterizes the therapist's stance in open-ended therapy. The teacher who does not encourage creative thinking among students about briefer applications of a psychoanalytic model may be discouraging students from doing the same when they are confronted with real-world decisions about how to accommodate their psychoanalytic sensitivities to the demands of the market. An additional concern is that some students may lose whatever appetite for psychoanalytic work is whetted by a course in the absence of being able to see its practical implications for clinical work in a market increasingly sensitive to the need for short-term therapy.

By encouraging creative applications of the model, including making client perceptions of the limits of the relationship a realistic issue in the treatment, the teacher can help students think about finding a place for psychoanalytic practice in managed care. In this regard, hypothetical case material developed specifically to address managed care issues that the psychoanalytic psychotherapist may have to confront can assist students in thinking through such dilemmas. By bringing this type of awareness to the course, the teacher addresses student concerns in a way that acknowledges contemporary practice issues while not minimizing the enduring value of long-term psychoanalytic treatment.

Field Sites

A second issue facing the teacher involves the relevance of the psychoanalytic model for graduate school training rotations. For instance, many clients seen by students in outpatient clinics as part of training rotations may not be ideal candidates for psychoanalytic treatment. Clients with dual diagnoses, severe personality disorders, or schizophrenia may be inclined to feel comfortable in either a more manifestly supportive or a problem-focused therapy approach. In addition, many of the settings in which students do their training may not be set up to provide the type of holding environment that helps make analytic therapy work. Cheifetz (1984) and Vlosky (1984) have provided telling accounts of the challenges that confront the analytically oriented student-trainee who seeks to set up a predictable therapy environment within a clinic setting. Moreover, there may be times when the student is interested in working psychoanalytically, but the clinical supervisor is not comfortable supervising within the analytic paradigm.

The teacher can be supportive of these concerns by encouraging students to seek out training sites where the supervisor is sensitive to the needs of a trainee motivated to apply psychoanalytic principles, is comfortable supervising psychoanalytic therapy, and is able to identify clients who may benefit from working with a student interested in applying psychoanalytic ideas to psychotherapy case work. It is under these conditions that the student is most likely to have a positive experience when learning about how to conduct a psychoanalytically informed therapy. Students who are inclined toward an analytic approach but who do not secure the aforementioned field site requisites may, on the other hand, find themselves working hard to develop rationalizations for the application of alternative treatment modalities, but being depressed over limited opportunities to learn more about the psychoanalytic model.

CLINICAL SEMINAR

The role of the clinical seminar in an academic setting, be it a seminar in psychotherapy or psychological testing, presents a special type of teaching challenge for the educator with psychoanalytic interests. Unlike other classes, a seminar is typically organized around a case presentation and discussion format, with students sharing clinical material and commenting, along with the teacher, on the quality of each other's work. Although the faculty member who leads a seminar may also teach several didactic courses, teaching a seminar requires a shift in style and content.

This shift in style and content is mandated by the focus on case application, student presentations, and integration of didactic content with real clinical situations. In a seminar, the teacher has an opportunity to help students think through real clinical dilemmas by illustrating proper technical application, by reasoning through a diagnostic issue, or by highlighting ethical issues as they arise in the context of casework. In addition to the teacher's input, other students share their experiences by comparing and contrasting the fit between the case being presented and their own fieldwork.

Because a seminar involves students' sharing clinical experiences with each other, often for the first time as part of the training program and with someone with whom they may have taken a didactic course, it arouses some unique vulnerabilities. Students and teachers see each other in a different light. In a seminar, students have an opportunity, and are usually required, to demonstrate their skills in the presence of peers and the teacher.

The teacher who leads a seminar by offering input on case material and facilitating discussion among group members has to deal with the theme of student and teacher anxieties about latent content implications of case material. Embedded within this theme are issues related to the teacher's identifications with the student who presents a case. These issues include (1) unconscious perceptions of student as classroom teacher, (2) countertransference in seminar leaders, and (3) competitive issues with clinical field supervisors.

Student as Teacher

Of utmost import to the clinical seminar teacher is the creation of an atmosphere in which students feel safe enough to share their work with their peers and the teacher. The case vignette offered in Chapter 5 illustrates some of the dilemmas that may confront a student who is making a case presentation. Ideally, the teacher contributes to a positive classroom experience for the presenter by being supportive, respectful, sensitive to group dynamics, and appropriately critical of student strategies for working with clients in a way that eases the student's ability to integrate this input.

The teacher's ability to mediate a safe space for the presenter is necessary because of the vulnerability to which the presenter is exposed when offering case material to a group for review. On the surface it may even appear that the student who presents a case for review has something in common with the teacher who lectures to a class. Both take pride in their work, share it with a group, receive criticism about their performance, and are vulnerable to narcissistic injury. This surface commonality, however, may be misleading.

In actuality, a clinical seminar differs in some important ways from the regular classroom. Unlike the formality of the usual classroom setting, a seminar is part clinic, part classroom, part supervision, and at times part therapy. Students who present cases in a seminar typically have not attained the same level of mastery over their clinical cases as have teachers over their course subject matter. Whereas teachers may have spent many years accumulating their knowledge base, most students are at a point in skill development where ongoing case supervision is needed.

As a result, students come to a seminar seeking knowledge and support.

Classroom teachers may find student input to be a rich and welcome source of ongoing stimulation and support that enhance their expertise. However, the teacher has presumably attained expertise, whereas students have not reached this level. Moreover, student performance is graded in a way that differs from student evaluations of teacher performance. It may be harder for a student to shrug off a weakness in clinical readiness than for a teacher to dismiss a few negative evaluations among an otherwise reasonably positive assessment by a group of students. Even if the teacher tends to be overly sensitive to the opinions in student evaluations, the reality consequences may be less harsh for the teacher than for the student. A poor evaluation by a field site supervisor, for example, can be a traumatic experience for a student, who must deal with departmental and personal consequences that result from inadequate performance on placement. Thus, students are understandably vulnerable when presenting their work. A low grade or an unfavorable assessment of skill level can hinder a student's progress through a mental health training program.

Being mindful of these differences between teacher-lecturer and student-presenter can help the teacher safeguard against projecting onto the student his or her own fantasies about presenting work to a large group. Failure to monitor these fantasies can lead the teacher to unwittingly perceive the student as teacher. The likelihood of such perceptions is intensified precisely because the seminar format tends to be more relaxed and colloquial than is the traditional classroom setting. It is this type of relaxed atmosphere, where students and teacher review process notes or listen to audio recordings of sessions, that stimulates the emergence of what may be otherwise dormant self-perceptions. For instance, teacher perceptions of students that are positive in tone and image lend themselves to the development of a supportive learning atmosphere. In contrast, perceptions that are disturbing can promote an unfavorable learning climate. Inevitable outcomes of such perception are disruptions in the teacher's ability to maintain an appropriately instructive stance when relating to students.

Countertransference in Seminar Leaders

Watkins (1985) has presented four types of identification that can signal countertransference reactions in therapists. These countertransference identifications can be applied to the relationship between seminar teacher and student. In each situation, the teacher's sensitivity to countertransference reactions can enhance the quality of the seminar student's development and deepen the teacher's appreciation of his or her own dynamics in the traditional classroom setting.

Overprotective Countertransference

The teacher is overly solicitous of the student. Such solicitation takes the form of viewing the student as fragile and in need of protection. As a result, the teacher feels uneasy with perceptions of the student's vulnerability. This type of identification with a student, which speaks on one level to the teacher's own hypervalent need for support, may be exemplified by the teacher's answering a challenging question posed by another student in the seminar rather than letting the presenter answer the question. In this case, the teacher protects the student from what the teacher perceives as the student's frailty. Unconsciously, however, the teacher may be signaling his or her own fear of being challenged by students. Another way in which the teacher's own need for protection from potentially disruptive fantasies may be enacted in the seminar is by being overly supportive, to the detriment of encouraging the student's introspection. In this situation, the teacher may hinder the student's progress by not fostering self-exploration. Instead, the teacher may direct the student to a reading, offer a hypothesis about the student's handling of a case, or revise significant portions of a test report in a manner that excuses the student and does not foster a sense of independent responsibility for clinical judgments. Similar to the first scenario, the teacher in this situation may be indicating his or her own need for external supports and underlying anxiety around being critiqued in the classroom.

Benign Countertransference

The teacher experiences a strong need to be liked by a particular student or fears that a particular student will react angrily if criticized. Such reactions to students may reflect aspects of the teacher's identification with the presenter and arouse fantasies of being challenged by students when presenting material to a class in the traditional lecture format. In this case, the need to be liked by a few students may create difficulty for the teacher who refrains from offering critique when such critique is in fact warranted (Goldsmith 1994, Kane et al. 1994). For example, because of a seminar teacher's need to be liked by a student, the teacher may decide to avoid any discussion creating fantasized discomfort for the student around transference and countertransference issues that have arisen in the student's casework. This tactic ultimately limits the learning opportunities for both the student and his or her classmates. Rather than address these issues, the teacher may encourage the student to apply certain techniques that are actually incongruent with the way in which the teacher would direct most other students under similar conditions. By taking this approach, the seminar leader is able to minimize the fantasy of unsettling a specific student and therefore strengthen the fantasy of being liked by that student, but at a cost to the student's educational experience.

Rejecting Countertransference

The seminar leader takes a punitive stance with students who present as needy or dependent. Underlying anxieties of the seminar leader may include a fear of being the object of what is felt as a student's demandingness or a fear of taking any responsibility for the student's development. In this situation, the seminar leader may fail to intervene when needed, thereby letting a needy student flounder in the relative absence of support or fostering an atmosphere where other students unite to voice overly critical remarks to the student who is presenting. Analog scenarios in the traditional classroom may include teachers who do not respond to student questions in a timely manner or who encourage students to seek answers on their own, without providing appropriate guidance either through verbal intervention or through citing important resource material.

Hostile Countertransference

In this situation there is an open dislike for a particular student, a dislike marked by aggressive exchanges. The seminar leader may be unnecessarily confrontational, badgering, or otherwise openly disrespectful of a student's efforts. For example, the seminar leader may brush aside a student's initial effort to interpret transference–countertransference dynamics by devaluing the student's work or demean a student's psychodiagnostic formulations of a difficult case without sensitivity to the student's phenomenology as presenter. Such teacher reactions in a seminar can signal inappropriate reactions by the teacher in traditional classroom settings; such reactions take the form of devaluing student input, admonishing alternative viewpoints, and deriving gratification from student struggles.

In each of these four types of identification, the seminar leader is in a position to potentially impede student progress. Through appropriate use of self-analytic strategies, however, the seminar leader can become increasingly aware of specific tendencies toward certain types of students and use this awareness to enhance the atmosphere of the clinical seminar.

Competition with Clinical Supervisors

The seminar leader has the responsibility of listening to and critiquing student presentations. It is through this role that the seminar leader makes important contributions to student skill development. The faculty status of the seminar leader implies a certain expertise, thereby arousing the fantasy in students that the seminar leader has all of the answers. The fact that the seminar leader also gives grades may make it hard for certain students to take a reasonably objective stance when evaluating the quality of input that is offered by the seminar leader.

Students may at times find themselves confused about whether to follow the directives of the seminar leader or the field site supervisor. Indeed, it is not unusual for students to sense an underlying competition between the site supervisor and the seminar leader. The seeds for such competition are clearly sown by the presence of two experienced clinicians with authority to influence case formulation.

There are, however, at least two important ways in which the seminar leader is likely to differ from the field site supervisor. The seminar leader's awareness of each distinction can help safeguard against the emergence of competition with the field site supervisor. The first difference can be tied to structural distinctions between clinical supervision and classroom-oriented seminars in relation to liability. The student's primary clinical supervisor often resides outside the university or college setting, selects cases for the student, and monitors client progress. The clinical supervisor offers regular input and holds ultimate responsibility for the case (Bennett et al. 1990, Cormier and Bernard 1982, Harrar et al. 1990). Comments offered to a student by peers or by the teacher in a seminar may carry some clout, but their application must ideally receive the supervisor's endorsement lest case control lie in the hands of people who have no direct ties to the client.

Second, clinical case material, unlike classroom lecture material, is often highly charged with rich interpersonal dynamics that address sensitive issues in the student's personal life. A positive supervisory relationship that accrues trust during individual weekly meetings may allow some room for the student's disclosure of personal material in a way that enhances case understanding. Seminar presentations, in contrast, are often one-shot deals. Students may present once or twice a semester to a group of individuals with whom they have some familiarity, but the type of interpersonal momentum that breeds intimate personal disclosures may not occur in the seminar format. Some students, for example, may say very little during a full year in a seminar save for the time that they present a case, with class protocol providing the group seminar leader with few means for drawing out individual students who display anxious, oppositional, or self-conscious features.

The seminar leader's appreciation of these two differences serves the student in several ways. First, the seminar leader is apt to encourage the student to present all recommendations made in the seminar to the site supervisor for review. This type of communication displays sensitivity to the student's relationship with the supervisor and also conveys an image of the seminar leader that is supportive and respectful of appropriate lines of authority. Second, the seminar leader is able to use differences in case responsibility vis-à-vis the site supervisor as a way of teaching students about ethics and liability issues in relation to case management. For instance, the seminar leader can highlight the importance of checking first with a supervisor before introducing a new technique with a client. By directing the student to check first with the immediate supervisor, the seminar leader encourages a collaborative professional relationship in which the authority of the supervisor is accorded full respect and demonstrates a sensitivity to the liability risk of making clinical decisions about case management in the absence of the authority to do so. Explaining both points to the student has clear instructional benefit. Third, the seminar leader is able to maintain appropriate classroom boundaries and disengage from a possible desire to forge quasi-therapeutic relationships with students that may be inappropriate for a large group in an academic setting.

Fourth, by being mindful of distinctions between leading a seminar and conducting supervision, the seminar leader is in a good position to alert students to a tendency on their part to draw seminar leader and site supervisor into competition with each other. For example, the seminar leader who keeps clear boundaries around case management and is able to refer critical issues presented in a seminar to the site supervisor can help the student see how he or she may be pitting teacher and supervisor against each other. This situation may take the form of a student's annoyance over what are perceived as conflicting directives from the teacher and the site supervisor. The teacher who is not overly invested in taking control of the case is able to redirect the student to the supervisor to further process the potential risks and benefits of assisting a client in a particular way.

PART III

THE PSYCHODYNAMICS OF TEACHING TASKS

CHAPTER 8

Preparation

Preparation for a course or a class is a fundamental teaching activity that taps different facets of the teacher's scholarship and interpersonal skill. Teachers set aside blocks of time in order to prepare for classes in anticipation of creating an instructional format that is conducive to student learning and inquiry. Typically, preparation includes reading various writings in order to identify critical topics within a specific area, reviewing previous course evaluations, outlining lectures, replacing old material with updated scholarship, and developing examinations.

In addition to being a scholarly activity, the preparation of either an academic course or a specific class represents an ongoing clinical task for the psychoanalytically informed teacher. Preparing to teach, like undertaking any other teaching pursuit, requires interest, desire, and a vision of making a difference in the lives of students. Because the course content is tied to the teacher's life experiences and value system, however, preparation necessarily becomes an interpersonal enterprise with dynamic implications. Data for classroom preparation may evolve, for instance, from the teacher's clinical work as both client and therapist, analysis of dreams, the intimacies and intricacies of significant attachments, familiarity with a body of literature within his or her discipline, previous experience as a student, prior teaching experiences with the same and other courses, student need, departmental considerations, institutional demand, and time constraint. For the teacher who has a strong psychoanalytic interest, preparation is an ongoing process.

On either the macrolevel of organizing a full course or the microlevel of outlining a specific lecture, preparation draws the teacher close to psychoanalytic concepts. The dynamics of preparation make this encounter unavoidable. Teachers who are attuned to the dynamics of preparation readily sense the mobilization of psychological resources in anticipation of the intrapsychic and interpersonal nuances associated with preparation. Different preparation styles notwithstanding, manifestation of dynamic processes is a thread common to the preparation process.

I have chosen not to separate the dynamics of preparing for a course from the preparation of a single lecture or series of lectures within the larger course. There are six general areas that can place preparation within a psychoanalytic model: (1) preparation as clinical process; (2) regression and creativity in classroom preparation; (3) the teacher's identifications with teacher role models, (4) the teacher's character trends; (5) students as inner voice; and (6) administrators as inner voice.

PREPARATION AS CLINICAL PROCESS

The type of preparation that underscores the teacher's work emanates from dynamic processes with which the psychoanalytic therapist may be familiar. If preparation is defined as the readiness to teach and if teaching can be

understood as a clinical activity, then similarities between
the processes that mediate the experience of therapist and
teacher can be identified across several borders. For both
teacher and therapist, preparation is an open-ended process that traverses developmental stages, is subject to
improvisation, and involves identifications, regressions,
formulations, and commitments.

Preparation as a Therapy Analog

The process that denotes an analytically oriented therapy
has a beginning, middle, and end stage in which there are
no finite boundaries that differentiate way stations. To be
sure, therapy does have chronological start and stop
points, but time demarcation in the unconscious is far less
reliable than is its conscious correlate. Indeed, the same
issues that surfaced at the start of therapy may again
ascend to prominence as therapy winds down. Moreover,
the intensive work done during the middle phase of
treatment, while anchored in its beginning, is both
precipitant to its ending and revisionistic to its past. For
example, if therapy is initiated in response to the ending
of a significant relationship in which the client perceived
himself or herself as having been unwittingly victimized,
then the ending of therapy will probably be colored by an
intensification of the same personality characteristics and
interpersonal paradigms that were subject to modification
through therapy, especially during the middle phase of
the treatment. The client should now be more insightful,
however, about these same paradigms, be able to work
with them with greater facility and maturity, and
understand their historical moorings in a manner different
from the level of understanding that operated at the
beginning of therapy. Throughout the treatment, the
therapist formulates material, revises and refines clinical

impressions, and examines his or her commitment to the client by both monitoring and working with transference and countertransference reactions. Although therapy has a formal ending, client and therapist will continue to reflect privately on the nature of their relationship long after they have ceased meeting.

Although different in content, the teacher's preparation can be conceptualized within the same genre of parameter that shapes the therapist's work. First, similar to the therapist's identification of salient client conflicts at the onset of treatment, teachers must also articulate at the onset of the course the central issues with which students need help. These issues are represented by the topics outlined in course syllabi. The teacher, functioning here along quasi-therapeutic lines, uses his or her judgment of student educational needs in making determinations about which topics to address. As the teacher moves through the course, there are reactions to students that result in modification of initial impressions concerning student need. These reactions may produce adjustments to the tempo of lectures, defensiveness, or insights gleaned from student questions. All such reactions have the potential of impeding, stalling, or facilitating the quality of subsequent lectures and the receptiveness of students to lecture content. In this regard, reactions, too, bear kinship to the type of therapist reactions that influence the progress of clients in therapy. The teacher's ability to balance structure with flexibility, much like the therapist's ability to work creatively within a psychoanalytic paradigm, is central to empathic and responsive instruction (Ebel 1988). Lastly, termination of a class, not unlike the ending of therapy, does not necessarily represent the discontinuation of the relationship between student and teacher. Instead, the reciprocity of influence that characterizes this relationship continues to impact impressions of teaching and learning well beyond ending dates.

REGRESSION AND CREATIVITY IN
CLASSROOM PREPARATION

Teaching clinical content to mental health students is a creative venture that can also be understood in light of regressive phenomenona. The teacher who can bridge clinical and nonclinical contexts across an experiential continuum and who can work with his or her own experiences creatively, is able to do so because of a capacity for controled psychological regression. Regression here entails a relaxation of typical ideational defenses in the service of deepening one's experiential involvements in teaching relationships. Regression involves the teacher's relationship to subject matter in a way that includes heightening the three psychological processes of immersion, vulnerability, and criticality.

Immersion as a Regressive Phenomenon

In order to invest emotionally in the preparation process, the teacher needs to give up a degree of cognitive control. The gradual relaxation of cognitive controls that issue from an intense involvement in the didactic subject matter allows for the creation of rich examples, vignettes, and explanations that are integrated within the fabric of clinical and life experiences. Much like the client who is able to give responses without excessive guardedness during a Rorschach test, the classroom teacher who prepares for teaching through immersion in the richness of literature and life experience that shape preparation also yields a rich protocol.

The teacher's regressive absorbtion when preparing course material can therefore be understood on one level as a response to becoming immersed in the material that will be taught to students. Immersion reflects not only a

preoccupation with the subject under study, but an experiential connection to the unconscious implications of the
subject matter. Although not manifestly obvious, a teacher's interest in specific or varied subjects can be understood as immersion in the service of unconscious mastery
strivings. The teacher develops an empathic bond with
ideas and with the characters portrayed in vignettes.

Through this type of empathy, the teacher studies not
only the written word, but what the written word says
about the teacher. For example, the teacher who is committed to such topics as severe psychopathology, countertransference, and research design as instructional areas
ostensibly spans varied dimensions of psychological
boundary ranging from the raw phenomenology of schizophrenia to the regulated fluctuations descriptive of countertransference to the orderly management of psychologies
through quantitative methodology. Intense investments in
specific topics afford proximity to disturbing material
while both regulating and neutralizing type and intensity of
contact. Being able to locate oneself in readings, or reading
in order to search oneself out, is, therefore, a regressive
experience that permits identifications with clinical material that allow the teacher to integrate and translate ab-
stractions to students.

Vulnerability and Criticality as Regressive Phenomena

The immersive quality of classroom preparation brings
into salience several psychological features, among them
vulnerability and criticality. Later in this chapter I discuss
how different personality styles embody psychological
features that are intensified during preparation and that
can either enhance or detract from the teacher's preparation experience. The way in which a hysterical personality
manifests criticality may, for example, be different from

the manner in which criticality is manifested by the depressive personality. Character style notwithstanding, however, the teacher's immersion in a body of knowledge in the context of scholarly preparation to teach heightens psychological vulnerability and arouses psychological criticality.

Vulnerability

The teacher's psychological vulnerability is increased because of the constant presence of potentially conflictual psychological material. Whether thinking about the course, reading material for the next class, outlining a lecture, or fantasizing about an examination format, the teacher keeps close contact with course content and its unconscious implications. For instance, the process of developing a clinical vignette about a client with borderline personality organization, preparing a Rorschach protocol that reflects narcissistic pathology, or critiquing an article about parallel processes and countertransference in supervision may engage the teacher in ways that trigger the recall of, or reflection on, disquieting events in his or her own personal experience.

The teacher's involvement with clinical material and the concomitant vulnerability to which this involvement exposes the teacher has a double edge. On the one hand, it affords the teacher an opportunity to develop a higher level of understanding of the material that may be symbolically tied to conflict. For example, preparation may conjure up recollections of a very difficult client or an uncomfortable supervisory experience that the teacher must now organize conceptually as part of developing course material. Here the teacher uses the preparation process as an opportunity to strengthen mastery strivings by imposing concepts on what may have been previously experienced as a predominantly affect-laden database.

Both the imposing of concepts and the distance from which the teacher now can reexamine old events afford revisionistic perspectives for grasping deeper meanings from significant incidents in the teacher's own professional development. On the other hand, the teacher must still confront the unsettling residue of this same database. Thus, in the midst of a felt sense of vulnerability exists a chance for a more mature understanding of the conflictual events that occurred at an earlier point in the teacher's development.

Criticality

In addition to the possibility of being on shaky terrain at different phases of the preparation process, the teacher's criticality may also become rigid in response to teasing out conceptual and experiential essence from irrelevance. That which would otherwise be ignored now becomes the object of intensive scrutiny as the teacher searches both the literature and his or her own personal experience for clarity, accuracy, and relevance in deciding what to teach and how to teach it. Both new and old literature are reviewed with an eye toward contemporary applications, quality of fit, historical implication, and ease with which students can understand the written word.

During this search the teacher may also become aware of certain limitations within his or her own knowledge base. The teacher may experience rivalrous feelings toward those individuals who have made a significant contribution to a particular body of knowledge in which the teacher also has a personal investment. In other cases, the teacher may pull back from criticality by seeing the good in all and may pile the reading list high. In short, the way that different teachers address issues related to discrimination of course material may in part reflect the symbolic implications of the material under review.

THE TEACHER'S IDENTIFICATIONS WITH
TEACHER ROLE MODELS

Among the most prominent variables influencing preparation are the teacher's identifications with professional role
models, including previous teachers, supervisors, and
therapists. It is hard to discern their specific impact on the
teacher's work, but the fact that the teacher has learned
something about organization, timely revision, and tempo
from each of them suggests some common thread to their
contribution to the teacher's classroom preparation. In
this context, the teacher's identifications permit ongoing
attachments to those professionals who have impacted the
teacher and made a difference in his or her work as
clinician and teacher. Identificatory processes operate
through the provision of internal regulatory functions
over the teacher's interests, attitudes, and style in the
classroom. A review of the teacher's identifications with
prior teachers helps to further clarify the way in which
these identifications influence disposition toward classroom preparation.

The Teacher's Prior Teachers

Students who eventually become teachers are influenced
in this direction by experiences with their own teachers.
Internal dialogue that defines the teacher's relationship to
prior teachers in relation to preparation includes such
commentary as: "What did I like about the way he taught
this course?" "What was it about her examinations that
really made me think?" "I remember a teacher I had who
used to create anxiety when . . . . What can I do differently for my students?" "I want my students to read what
I read when I was a student in this same course." "I never

want my students to have the type of experience that I had when . . . ."

Ideally, positive identifications with prior teachers dominate the teacher's internal world. In such cases, there exists a predominance of introjective imagery in which the student experiences the teacher as insightful, poised, creative, patient, and accessible across interactions. The student who later becomes a teacher has these images upon which to draw when preparing a course. As such, preparation will take on an analytically oriented tack characterized by the teacher's patient and deliberate approach to a rich body of data in the service of developing an empathic connection to students.

In cases in which there may not be a predominance of positive teaching introjects to gently guide the preparation process, the teacher may prepare by dictum. Such preparation involves rigid perspectives on education that display minimal resonance with student need. Manifestation of such rigidity may include the teacher's firm adherence to examination methods that are modeled on authoritarian approaches to learning. Teachers who are disposed toward rigid approaches to preparation, lecturing, and examination remain distant from other data that may make the course more engaging to students.

THE TEACHER'S CHARACTER TRENDS

The teacher's character trends represent another source of data from which an understanding of classroom preparation can be developed. The uniqueness of the teacher's personality style and the salience of selective character traits within that style operate unconsciously and leave their mark on the overall quality of the teacher's preparation. For instance, teachers with compulsive personality features are likely to prepare a course differently from teachers whose compulsivity is not a particularly key feature in their personality structure. Compulsivity may lead one teacher to the brink of exhaustion in searching out an entirety of literature, whereas a less compulsive approach to preparation may result in fewer references but also in fewer sleepless nights.

Four character styles that are grounded in psychoanalytic personality theory (Kernberg 1975, Lerner 1991, Shapiro 1965) may have an adaptive or a maladaptive impact on the teacher's preparation. These character styles are obsessive-compulsive, hysterical, depressive, and narcissistic.

Obsessive-Compulsive Style

The presence of an obsessive-compulsive personality can be an asset to the teacher's preparation. The scrupulous, ruminative, detached, critical, perfectionistic, conscientious, compliant, orderly, and dutiful approaches that denote features of the obsessive-compulsive style all have adaptive implications for teacher preparation. Careful attention to the details of planning, thorough and critical review of the literature, and concern with correctness, accuracy, and accountability all factor into successful preparations.

Potential liabilities of the obsessive-compulsive personality can make the preparation process uncomfortable for the teacher. Rigid positions about what to teach, limited resonance with student needs, and a dispassionate approach toward subject matter grounded in human relationships all work against the type of preparation that lends itself to empathic teaching. For example, the teacher with a rigid obsessive-compulsive style may become bogged down in endless rumination over the order in which certain lecture topics should be presented. The salience of perfectionistic features may lead to continual faultfinding with research and clinical work portrayed in case illustrations; in such instances, enthusiasm for teaching is dampened by the weight of a harsh inner voice. Workmanlike efforts may deteriorate into unending projects in which relationships suffer at the expense of rigid personality characteristics. If rigidity is excessive, then classroom performance will probably receive negative feedback on student evaluations and place the teacher with obsessive-compulsive features in the uncomfortable position of possibly having to defend himself or herself to administrative authority.

Hysterical Style

In contrast to the ideational bent of the obsessive-compulsive character, individuals with predominantly hysterical personalities operate more from a base of emotionality. Salient personality features include impressionism, sensitivity, sociability, suggestibility, and seductiveness. There is a playful, engaging, and warm quality that distinguishes the hysterical personality from the more reserved and controlled obsessive-compulsive. On a continuum, hysterical personality features also manifest in ways that facilitate or impede preparation.

From the standpoint of adaptation, the hysteric's approach to preparation is likely to be more relaxed and spontaneous than overly disciplined; things will get done, but they need not proceed along the lines of a fixed plan. Because of the hysteric's sensitivity to mood and tempo, lecture topics may be open to revision across semesters, rather than remain unchanged even when change may be warranted. There may also be a willingness to try alternative approaches to instruction, an attitude that issues from empathy to student need and receptiveness to feedback.

The adverse consequences of rigid hysterical features

for teacher preparation may manifest in several ways. For example, a relaxed approach to preparation may degenerate into forgetfulness that masks an underlying noncompliant attitude. Examinations are developed in which grading criteria are highly impressionistic and lack the degree of specificity that allows for easy justification of grades. Efforts to involve students in shaping course direction through solicitation of ongoing feedback may slip into an unstructured mode in which students begin to feel uncomfortable about the teacher's apparent laissez-faire approach to classroom instruction. All such considerations may result in unfavorable course evaluations that disappoint teachers, students, and administrators.

Depressive Style

The depressive personality style is characterized by a disposition toward self and others in which sensitivity to loss and rejection, guilt, tendency toward self-deprecation, and pessimism tend to dominate. There is an air of seriousness to the depressive character that bears similarity to the disposition of the obsessive-compulsive but differs from the upbeat tenor of the hysterical character. Compared to obsessive-compulsive, however, the depressive character is more easily attuned to interpersonal dynamics and is less likely to operate under the pressure of perfectionistic strivings.

Adaptive features of the depressive style in relation to teacher preparation include sensitivity to students, seriousness in teaching attitude, appreciation of realistic limitations of knowledge imposed by a body of literature, self-criticism, and a willingness to make changes in the direction of a course based on student feedback. The depressive character, because of his or her embedment within a relational fabric, may also have the advantage of being able to access rich meaning from clinical illustrations that supplement classroom presentation. With a ready sensitivity to interpersonal nuance and loss, the teacher with depressive personality traits remains ever close to the types of clinical issues that attract students and is able to use this sensitivity in organizing lectures, projects, and tests that engage students empathically.

In contrast to these facilitative qualities, the maladaptive expression of depressive personality poses potential problems for classroom preparation. For example, punitive self-reprimand along the lines of nothing being good enough for students, difficulty moving beyond an unproductive pessimism about the relevance of what will be taught, excessive undoing in response to student complaints about examination grades, and a thin-skinned reaction to the type of criticism that students occasionally give teachers all bode unfavorably for different facets of preparation. The intensification of depressive personality features renders the teacher susceptible to an irritating moodiness that rankles individuals who impose their needs upon the teacher and that can make the prospect of teaching, and being taught, unrewarding.

Narcissistic Style

Of the four personality styles represented in this section, the predominance of narcissistic features is potentially the most disruptive to teacher preparation and student welfare. Although theoretical debates offer different points of view on the determinative factors in the development of a narcissistic style, there is a general consensus about the salience of particular personality traits. Central to the narcissistic style are an inflated sense of self-esteem, an exquisite vulnerability to slights, a tendency toward devaluations or idealizations of others, an expectation that interpersonal entitlements will be forthcoming regardless of effort, a susceptibility to aggressive or depressive episodes, and a shallow emotionality.

Yet these traits may not be easily visible on a regular basis. For example, under optimal conditions in which self-esteem is not perceived as being at risk, narcissistic traits may remain muted in their intensity and attractive interpersonally. In these situations, the teacher with narcissistic personality features may be perceived as being poised, engaging, magnetic, and in control. Students may find themselves drawn to the teacher, and the teacher may perceive himself or herself as having a magical touch.

The disturbing dimensions of narcissistic personality attributes are most likely to emerge in response to specific threats to self-esteem. If for some reason the teacher feels threatened, for example, when an administrator has become privy to complaints about the teacher's apparent arrogance and cold reaction to genuine student concerns, then the teacher's narcissistic defenses may rigidify. Such rigidification may lead the teacher to act out conflicts with students and administrators around the experience of preparation. For example, changes in syllabi that detract from student learning may occur at whim and without regard to impact on students. Examinations may be constructed with vindictive intent. Perceptions of negative feedback from students may result in the destabilization of grandiose self-imagery and lead to either depressive episodes in which work ethic declines or aggressive approaches that countermand any perceived challenge. The limited capacity of the narcissistic character to empathize with students leaves little room for the type of responsiveness to critical feedback that ultimately enhances teaching and learning.

STUDENTS AS INNER VOICE

The teacher's classroom preparation cannot be separated from the inner voices of students. I am referring here to the teacher's fantasies about the ways in which students experience a particular course. These fantasies accompany all aspects of preparation. Although not articulated consistently in first-person dialogue, the teacher's fantasized images of students embrace the teacher's perceived competence and his or her audience. Two questions appear to capture the inner voices of students: Can I teach this? Whom am I teaching?

Can I Teach This?

This question speaks to the teacher's perceived level of competence within a given subject domain. For some teachers, this question is answered easily. They feel either self-confident or unsure of their ability to deliver the goods to students in a manner keeping with the level of expertise that students and administrators demand. Other teachers may feel more confident about part of a course but less comfortable with other material. For example, a teacher may have a strong grasp of, and commitment to, one neuropsychological test, but feel less strongly about a second such test that must also be taught to students as part of a course in neuropsychological assessment. If confronted with this situation, one teacher may forge ahead and initiate a self-instructional program in which efforts to develop higher degrees of mastery in the area of weakness would be the subject of remedial work. Another teacher may opt for the low road, dismiss the test outright or cover it cursorily through a handout, hesitate to invite a guest speaker because of a conflict around competition, and deprive students of an opportunity to gain familiarity with a particular psychological test. What the teacher chooses to teach or omit speaks volumes to the teacher's fantasized anticipation of student response.

Whom Am I Teaching?

The inner voices of students touch not only the teacher's own sense of skill but also the ability and interest levels of

students. Much in the same way that classroom preparation remains tied to the inner voices of students in relation
to the teacher's felt level of competency, so too is the
teacher's felt level of competency bound to student abili-
ties and interests. Throughout preparation, the teacher
may be responding to questions about whether class size is
optimal and the students equally skilled; whether the
course is basic or advanced, required or elective; and
whether the students issue from multiple disciplines or are
on the same degree track.

Topic selection or lecture foci are evaluated accordingly. If, for example, students on different degree tracks
within a single department are required to take a class
together, the teacher needs to be sensitive to the way the
course material may influence the different training needs
of students. Assignments that display sensitivity to these
needs are helpful to students and reflect the teacher's
sensitivity to the different learning requirements that operate in a heterogeneous class. Presenting the material
generically may provide the necessary foundation for
application within a discipline, but generic assignments
may not be able to provide students with the type of
specificity needed in order to tailor application to the
diverse populations that define disciplines.

In addition to considering the utility of course content
in relation to an academic discipline, the teacher's preparation must also take into account variance of student skill
level. Because adult education in mental health attracts
individuals from different chronological age groupings
and life experiences—including different levels of experience within the field of mental health—the teacher may
need to develop a course in a manner that finds a comfortable middle ground. How, for example, can students with
different entry-level skills be taught in a way that gives all
students the freedom to draw from their experiences
while the teacher remains sensitive to obvious discrepancies across experience levels? By engaging students in

active dialogue throughout the preparation process, the teacher remains better equipped to address these types of questions with integrity, sensitivity, and conscientiousness.

ADMINISTRATORS AS INNER VOICE

Another internal voice that accompanies the teacher's preparation is the collective voice of academic administrators. By virtue of their authority in the instructional domain, administrators stimulate the teacher's superego deliberations around different aspects of classroom preparation. Perception of academic freedoms notwithstanding, teachers must still remain mindful of their relationship to administrators as part of their preparation. These relationships invariably color both the quality of instruction and student sentiment around learning.

In its most benign tone, the inner voice of administrators encourages and supports academic freedom within the parameters of the institutional mission; is trusting of faculty integrity; remains attentive to, but not constrained by, student concerns; and sets broad standards for academic excellence permitting the development of faculty and student scholarship through a variety of venues. Under these conditions, faculty are able to think creatively about preparation without feeling the types of excessive pressures around rigid conformity that exacerbate character trends as well as other components of the preparation process. Faculty in these contexts may therefore be more motivated to teach in new areas, less anxious about the impact of an occasional complaint about quality of instruction lodged by a student, and freer to encourage diversity of ideas in the service of higher-level integration. Things can change, however, if faculty perceive a harsh ness in the tone of administrative voice. Such harshness may resonate under the atypical circumstances mandating that all relevant course material, such as syllabi, readings, and examinations, be critiqued by an administrator before being given to students or that all complaints registered by students be processed initially through an administrator. Additional sources of faculty anxiety that may arise in response to administrative tenor include conscription to courses outside the scope of the teacher's interest and expertise, enrollment considerations necessitating modifications from preferred instructional format with little or no advance notice to the teacher, and unreasonable demands for scholarly contribution and productivity.

In sum, the teacher's preparation entails substantially more work than might be suggested by manifest observations that cast the teacher's preparation tasks within the frame of collating, reviewing, outlining, and time managing. Subsumed within these activities is an intensive dynamic process that shapes the direction of a course.

A teacher was placed on roster to teach a course that this teacher had not taught in several years. The teacher had a vague recollection of being approached many months ago about possibly being interested in again teaching this course "sometime in the future." The teacher had agreed to do so, but was taken aback that the course had been scheduled much sooner than expected.

Preparation was initiated ambivalently and on short notice. The teacher felt a bit out of step with the developments that had occurred recently in this field, but was still interested in the area and needed the course in order to meet academic credit load requirements. Having previously taught this course, the teacher looked at the old evaluations; they were essentially positive, save for a few comments that the teacher had not spaced the three class examinations adequately. Students had felt that the examinations were too close together and that they had not been given sufficient time to reflect on the feedback, recover from the examination experience itself, and then integrate the old material with whatever new material was presented as part of the cumulative nature of the course. The teacher took these comments to heart, recognized that they reflected the teacher's identification with the person who had taught this course to the teacher in graduate school, and promised to revise the examination format when planning the course.

In addition to the anxiety stirred by having to prepare a course on short notice, the teacher was also aware that a rumor had begun to circulate among faculty that course syllabi and lecture notes would be subject to random review by administrators. Administrators had voiced concern about teacher preparation in a memorandum circulated recently in which faculty were asked for "your full cooperation in this matter." Apparently, several students had taken to administration complaints about being assigned outdated reading material. A perception of a few faculty as being apathetic toward teaching was beginning to permeate administration in a way that raised anxiety among faculty as a whole. Although nothing about random review had been delineated in the administrative memorandum, there was a general consensus that such review could indeed occur and was within the parameters of administrative authority.

In response to anxiety emanating from the aforementioned sources, the teacher approached preparation with an attitude different from the one that might have marked more relaxed circumstances. In essence, the teacher's preparation became uncomfortably vigilant across all fronts. For example, the teacher conducted an exhaustive literature review and read articles well into the night; even articles that had only peripheral implications for the course were read. These articles consisted of readings that the teacher would otherwise have quickly dismissed as secondary to the main points of the course; under the increased sense of pressure surrounding the meanings attached to course preparation, however, the teacher decided to leave no stone unturned. More than the ordinary amount of weekend time was devoted to meticulous outlining of class notes; at one point, the teacher even had the fantasy of reading lectures from prepared texts, but squelched this idea because of its potential for distancing students. Ruminations about grading and excessive solicitation of class input around "the best" examination dates (on which no one could agree) rounded out the teacher's anxious reaction concomitant with classroom preparation.

From this example, it is relatively easy to see that the dynamics of classroom preparation extend much deeper than what is perceived from surface behaviors. Caught off guard by the seemingly sudden decision to schedule a course that the teacher had agreed to teach, the teacher felt that inadequate time had been allotted to preparation. The fact that the teacher agreed to teach the course and then did not follow up the apparent ambiguity with which the scheduling was set rested as much with the teacher's ambivalence about teaching as with the way in which the teaching assignment was presented. Intensification of certain character features in response to the perception of administrative mandate around quality of instruction also factored into the teacher's preparation. In this case, the teacher believed rumors that lecture notes might be reviewed by higher-ups and did not check the accuracy of this rumor. In addition, the teacher's sensitivity to previous course evaluations, coupled with the affrontive nature of having work double-checked, led to a quality of preparation that bordered on excessive.

Although this may be perceived as an extreme case designed to exaggerate an academic reality, such a scenario nevertheless offers insight into the subtlety of dynamics that can influence the teacher's classroom preparation. The teacher's desire to teach and learn, character trends, and reactions to students, previous teachers, and administrators interface with the process of preparation to make it a clinical task of high order for the psychoanalytic educator.

CHAPTER 9

Lecturing

Although there are many ways to teach students, lecturing is clearly the preferred mode of classroom instruction. According to Centra (1993), the lecture is the primary or only method used by more than 80 percent of college teachers. In commenting on the possible reasons for this preference, Ebel (1988) noted that the safety and security derived from formal lecture presentations may account for its continuing popularity as an instructional method.

On the other hand, whether the lecture is the most productive means of fostering the acquisition of knowledge is a debatable point. Brookfield (1990), for instance, commented that many teachers are acculturated into a teaching system that adheres to lecturing as the preferred mode of teaching, even if alternative teaching strategies engage student learning in a more dynamic way. The rigid practice of lecturing may have particular consequences for the adult student who brings rich life experience to education. Adult learners in mental health professions are ready to draw on their own experiences for didactic purposes and may feel distanced by an authority-centered pedagogic experience that minimizes opportunities to engage in the collaborative, self-directed endeavors marking the androgogic approach to adult learning (Cross 1991, Merriam and Cafferella 1991).

For the psychoanalytically oriented teacher, lecturing to students has rich dynamic implications. Because of the process-oriented training that defines psychoanalytic clinical work, the shift to a relational style that is directive and content driven necessitates a psychological adjustment for the classroom teacher with a psychoanalytic bent. Even clinical courses require a fairly heavy dose of lecture in order to get main points across to students. Only in seminars do students take the lead by presenting casework. Given the discrepancy between the directive nature of lecturing and the nondirective nature of analytic therapy, the psychoanalytically informed teacher clearly stands at an ill-defined crossroad when lecturing to a class.

A psychoanalytic perspective on lecturing as a teaching task may be gained by considering (1) lecturing as a psychoanalytic contrast; (2) lecturing as an empathic intervention; (3) the teacher's vulnerability as lecturer; (4) countertransference manifestations during a lecture; and (5) lecture content as an interpersonal trigger.

LECTURING AS A PSYCHOANALYTIC CONTRAST

When considering the psychodynamics of teacher as classroom lecturer, one must consider the meaning of *lecturing to people* relative to the manifestation of its opposite pole in a psychoanalytically informed psychotherapy, in which the therapist refrains from lecturing to people. Lecturing to people from a position of authority is fraught with underlying implications that may be quite unsettling both for the lecturer and for the people toward whom the lecture is directed. Teachers are expected to be knowledgeable in all areas pertaining to the topic under discussion and to be able to answer most, if not all, of the questions raised by inquisitive students. Listening to people, on the other hand, is the stance of the psychoanalytic practitioner and gives a hearing to those who need to be heard.

Indeed, it is through an appreciation for the interpersonal process in psychoanalytic psychotherapy juxtaposed to the role of the teacher as lecturer to students that an understanding of the dynamics of the classroom lecture takes on new meanings. Lecturing to students is inherently at odds with psychoanalytic clinical work in a few key ways and therefore poses an integrative challenge to the teacher of psychoanalytic persuasion. Two such points of departure illuminate this premise: (1) the directive nature of lecturing and (2) lecturing as a closed information system.

The Directive Nature of Lecturing

One of the hallmarks of psychoanalytic psychotherapy is the therapist's nondirective approach. The therapist is disinclined to educate, advise, or otherwise disturb the continuity of the client's comments. In the psychoanalytic model, the client leads and the therapist follows. The nondirective nature of the analytic approach becomes part of the therapist's professional signature when staking claim to a theoretical position.

Therapists who press clients into psychological positions do so at the risk of disrupting the gradual and natural unfolding of conflicts that become organized around the therapeutic relationship. Such interpersonal pressure promotes premature mobilization of the client's anxieties against perceptions of the therapist's imposed and unsolicited authoritative stance. Under these conditions, clients recoil, feel shaken, anxiously submit to the therapist's authority, or balk aggressively. In each unique situation, there is a change of tempo at the seeming behest of the therapist's felt sense of urgency.

In this regard, the interpersonal demands of classroom lecturing, because of the teacher's direct influence over the topics and the pace of the lecture, would appear to be antagonistic to the nondirective therapy approach of the psychoanalytic therapist. The teacher's listening style, readiness to respond to questions, and search for underlying meaning are different from the therapist's stance on each matter. For example, the therapist waits patiently for the client to develop material; the teacher actively brings content to bear on students. The therapist has freedom to desist from answering direct questions; the teacher responds directly. The therapist culls unconscious perceptions from manifest content; the teacher stays on the straight and narrow of secondary process thinking.

The move from classroom lecturer to clinician and from clinician back to classroom lecturer is protected in part by the different structure and tasks of each role. There is a sanctioning of the teacher's movement away from process when teaching and of the therapist's focus on process in treatment. Nevertheless, there still remains the crunch of interdisciplinary adjustment that can tax the teacher with psychoanalytic training. To be trained psychoanalytically is to be grounded in a relational stance that in some ways reverses the balance of power presumed to exist within the teaching relationship. The psychoanalytic therapist respects resistances, refrains from direction, and views the client as having ultimate authority or final say in determining both the content to be reviewed and the expertise to evaluate the therapist's learning. Because the teacher as lecturer must adopt positions that challenge these precepts of psychoanalytic training—it is the teacher who has the expertise, the evaluative power, and the clout to put diffident students on the spot and thus bypass student blocks to learning—the merits of the lecture process itself require the teacher's ongoing internal assessment.

Lecturing as a Closed Information System

A second way in which lecturing poses a challenge to the basic tenets of psychoanalytic therapy is in its structure as a closed information system. The process of psychoanalytic psychotherapy holds that anything goes. Clients can say what they want, and therapists must work creatively and therapeutically with what they get.

Lectures, however, start and stop at the teacher's behest. Interesting topics that engage student curiosity come to a halt in a brief time period. Topic content is fixed, disseminated, and phased out in order to make space for new ideas. Ideally, there is an orderliness to topic presentation that facilitates both mastery of content and transitions across topics. Topics build on each other in a cumulative manner that permits higher-level syntheses.

An orderly procession of lecture topics makes sense in the classroom, but runs against the natural grain of the free-associative process governing the distribution of content in psychoanalytic therapy. Psychoanalytic therapy is an open-ended system in which topics emerge spontaneously without regard for time. In contrast, the lecture moves at a pace regulated by the teacher. Students have some influence over timing and length of stay with a particular concept, but by and large the teacher is under time constraints to present specific topics within clearly delineated time parameters.

Never are the adverse consequences of moving quickly through lecture material more obvious than when students feel a sense of loss on the introduction of a new topic. For example, if a teacher has been discussing a topic that seems timely and relevant, students may have difficulty shifting to new material. The lecturer's premature termination of a topic that excites students, stimulates questions, fosters discussion, and touches inner dynamics in a meaningful way can lead to a lull in the classroom atmosphere. Students raise fewer questions, the teacher can hear his or her own echo amid the sudden staleness of the classroom, and a hollow void develops where enthusiasm reigned only moments ago. These lost opportunities to continue with interesting content would appear to symbolize the nature of the closed system that in part defines the classroom lecture.

LECTURING AS AN EMPATHIC INTERVENTION

The manner in which the teacher presents lectures to his or her students can reflect a sensitive understanding of student experience when receiving lecture material (Lubin and Stricker 1992). Teachers who are sensitive to timing, technique, and dosage—three aspects of a sensible psychoanalytic technical stance in therapy—offer students an opportunity to receive lectures empathically.

Empathic lecturing requires that the teacher have an understanding not only of his or her subject matter but of his or her subjects. While the teacher lectures, the students are busy at work. They listen, take notes, raise questions, and search for organization in the material. Students who ask the teacher to slow down, speed up, spend more time responding to questions, or repeat specific material and students who manifest an underlying anxiety about one student dominating the class by rolling their eyes or other nonverbal gesturing do so in the service of tempering the lecture pace and regulating the teacher. Moreover, such actions represent attempts to connect to the teacher and strengthen an empathic bond between lecturer and recipients.

Because students are exquisitely sensitized to the teacher's presence, minor rifts in the quality of communications from the teacher take on deep meanings that may go unnoticed or be swallowed by the structure and occasional rigid regimentation of the lecture process. Incidents that the teacher takes for granted may actually be speaking to student perception of the teacher's empathic lapse. For example, the teacher who routinely digresses from main topics may wind up with students whose class notes look scrambled. A review of notes may show an array of arrows expressing the maze of communication that students map out in order to track the teacher. Other similar observations, including doodlings or drawings in the margins (which themselves have symbolic meanings), can be understood as indicators of frustration at the teacher's not having given students appropriate guidance with regard to the direction of the lecture. Teachers who flood students with handouts, assign abstruse reading material without appropriate classroom discussion, or do not allow time for periods of integration before moving to another topic run the risk of not staying close to student phenomenology. In contrast, teachers who are able to hold an appropriate pace, handle student inquiry and frustration with relative patience, and build formative measures into the lecture process in order to assess student understanding create an empathic stance with students.

THE TEACHER'S VULNERABILITY AS LECTURER

Appelbaum (1972), writing on the psychology of scientific papers from a psychoanalytic perspective, drew attention to the apparent contrast between the self-aggrandizing motive that factors into the decision to present scientific work and the limitations of lecturing as a vehicle for exciting the masses. The disappointments lying in wait for the self-aggrandizing presenter, along with other potential psychological vulnerabilities to which the lecturer is exposed, bring an additional dimension to the dynamics of the classroom lecture. Such vulnerabilities are overstimulation of the grandiose self, and the challenge of containment.

Overstimulation of the Grandiose Self

In a way, the arrival, performance, and departure of the lecturer can be compared to a three-movement concerto. The lecturer is on center stage for the duration of his or her presentation. Because students have paid tuition in order to have a seat in class, there is an arousal of affect that precedes the lecturer's arrival. Such affect may be anxious, fearful, or depressive in content, but each affect state may be understood as being linked to the anticipation of beginning the class period and to wondering what the class holds for the student.

The lecturer is then at the disposal of his or her audience during the formal presentation, moving from idea to idea, at times as a soliloquy and at times as a response to audience request. There are instances in which the need to balance student inquiry with the presentation of content takes on the nature of a musical duet. Movement toward class closure brings performance reviews; some students may wish to stay late for individual contact, others may be piqued by what they felt was a less than stellar effort, and still others may hold opinion in abeyance. The lecture therefore puts the teacher in a special place in relation to his or her students. Rarely is the teacher's special skill and knowledge on similar display in front of such a potentially rapt audience. The lecture provides the teacher a forum to share and impart special skills and knowledge, gather kudos, develop a coterie of admirers, and wield influence. Further, the fact that semester-long classes meet weekly for upward of four months ensures the teacher ample time to develop a rich base of influence with his or her students.

The heightening of the teacher's specialness, however, also places the teacher in a precarious spot. The freedom to showcase teaching talents is a heady experience, fraught with its own potential minefields of traumatic reenactment. For with the elevation of student expectation comes the hope of change but also the fear of disappointment. Both the hope of being inspired to new heights of learning that students bring to the class and their fear of being disappointed by the teacher's performance can impinge on the teacher's capacity for containment.

The Challenge of Containment

Containment necessitates ongoing management of thoughts and feelings that occur in the context of observing, lecturing, and listening to students. For instance, a teacher who is on a roll in front of the class is speaking expertly about a topic in which she has an emotional investment. Out of the corner of her eye, the teacher observes one student whose facial expression suggests that this student is taking umbrage at something the teacher has said in the context of lecturing. The teacher then fields a question that poses a direct challenge to the main lecture premise and perceives a subtle hostility in the student's tone. Has the teacher touched on an area with which the student has conflictual personal associations? Is the student struggling with competitive issues that surface in response to perceiving the teacher as the expert in the limelight? Or is the teacher externalizing her own aggression because she enjoys being neither challenged nor usurped during a lecture? In each case, the teacher's ability to identify, process, and respond to the student requires balancing a mature, overt response to the skeptical query with the potentially chafing quality of internal dialogue stirred by the student's question.

COUNTERTRANSFERENCE MANIFESTATIONS DURING A LECTURE

A recurrent theme in this book has been the susceptibility of teachers to countertransference reactions toward their students. The previous example of the teacher's internal struggle with the student's challenging question illustrates the type of lecture dynamic that can stimulate vulnerability to countertransference in teachers. Teachers can also manifest their countertransference around grading by delaying the return of examination papers because of anxiety about having to deal with student reaction to grades or by failing to keep the class for the full period because of insecurity about not having covered all relevant subject matter.

Clearly, then, the classroom lecture is yet another part of the teacher's work that remains ripe for countertransference manifestation. Expressions of countertransference during a lecture can take numerous forms and shadings in addition to those noted above. Two common paths through which the lecturer can evidence countertransference during a lecture are talking down to students and selective attention to particular students.

Talking Down to Students

By talking down to students, I am referring to situations in which the teacher exhibits minimal sensitivity to student inquiry. Teachers who are perceived in this light come across as dismissive and uncaring. Although underlying conflicts around authority are at the center of this attitude, the teacher may remain unaware of their manifestation because of rigid rationalizations against the conscious experience of conflict. Some of the ways in which this attitude is conveyed to students include clipped answers to questions, harshness in response to a perception of students as not being attentive enough to generate questions around the lecture material, and a defensive lecture tone in which the teacher makes it clear that while questions will be tolerated, they are not welcomed.

Selective Attention to Particular Students

A second way in which the teacher's countertransference is manifested during a lecture is through selective attention to particular students. Selectively attending to certain students represents an attachment dilemma for the teacher. When the teacher is perceived as having either favorites or scapegoats, for example, students begin to feel that they have been cast into roles that issue from the teacher's own needs rather than from the needs of students. Although the teacher may be unaware of a propensity to acknowledge one student more frequently than others, a tendency to make extended eye contact with another student, a readiness to respond abruptly when yet another student asks questions, or a seductive quality with one or more students, the students do take notice of the teacher's disposition and begin to react accordingly. The teacher's selectivity can breed competition, ire, and disappointment in students, each of whom may desire the teacher's acceptance and affirmation. In the absence of insight into such matters, the teacher unwittingly detracts from the essence of the lecture and introduces potential conflict for students in their attachment to the teacher.

LECTURE CONTENT AS AN
INTERPERSONAL TRIGGER

If the content of a lecture is broadly defined to include all comments by either teacher or student in relation to a particular topic, then it is quite possible that lecture content itself may embody elements of unconscious communication from teacher to student or from student to teacher. Because of the highly interpersonal nature of didactic content in mental health training curricula, it is easy to appreciate how lecture content can trigger interpersonal associations unique to each student and teacher. Listening to or presenting a lecture can trigger thoughts and feelings about oneself in relation to others. Two ways through which these types of associations manifest are spontaneous interpersonal questions that students ask and sharing of interpersonal vignettes by the teacher. The content of a lecture can take on unconscious meaning that remains sensitive to the relationship between teacher and student.

Spontaneous Interpersonal Questions That
Students Ask

The content of the teacher's lecture is an interpersonal communication to students, touching them in unique ways that encourage both their silent exploration of the meaning of lecture material in their lives and overt expressions of curiosity about how to better understand the material that is being presented. Thus, when students ask the teacher to help them clarify something that the teacher has said about relationships, are they not also asking the teacher for help in better understanding themselves and significant others in their lives?

A brief review of the types of questions to which I am referring and their possible interpersonal meanings may help to clarify this point. For instance, why may a student decide to raise a question in class that relates to a topic covered three classes ago? Why now? What has transpired to make this student raise this question at this time? What can the teacher do to bring added meaning to the student's present understanding? Why does a student ask the teacher several follow-up questions about a lecture topic that deals with understanding transference but no other questions about any other material covered in the same course? Was there something in the case example presented in conjunction with the lecture that held a special meaning for the student and stimulated the need to know more about this particular area?

Not only do questions of this type speak to the lecture topic as an interpersonal trigger for the student's life outside of the class, but they also hint at possible underlying perceptions of the teacher. Student perceptions of the teacher represent an additional factor influencing both the decision to ask questions and the content of the questions that are asked. For example, was there an inflection in the teacher's voice that stirred the student's associations? And how may this tone relate to perceptions of the teacher? Does the student now feel more comfortable with the teacher and therefore able to raise a question that had been suppressed for three classes? Does the student notice something in the teacher's demeanor that suggests a greater readiness to handle questions pertaining to a certain topic now? Does this student typically ask questions only after another student in class expresses uncertainty, therefore drawing strength from the other student's confusion and willingness to raise a question with the teacher? Does the content of the question itself address an issue pertaining to the teacher? Answers to these questions reveal an underlying perception of a teacher that can make a difference in a student's ability to understand a topic on a personal level.

Sharing of Interpersonal Vignettes by the Teacher

The lecture topic also stirs conscious and unconscious associations in the teacher that relate to conflictual personal content. When talking about psychopathology, interpreting projective test material, supervising a clinical case, or generating discussion about transference, the teacher's own personal history remains on call. Like students who raise questions, teachers use the classroom as a forum for processing their own reactions to the lecture material.

One way of processing these reactions is through the sharing of clinical material. The psychoanalytically informed teacher who lectures in the emotionally charged arena of mental health invariably shares clinical vignettes with students. The vignettes may be disguised versions of the teacher's own clinical work that are offered spontaneously or hypothetical illustrations that have been developed specifically for didactic purposes for integration with the prepared lecture.

Ostensibly, the sharing of these vignettes serves to anchor concepts to clinical application. By bringing clinical material into the class, the teacher encourages students to think critically about the utility of concepts as organizers of development, psychopathology, and treatment. Spontaneous disclosures of clinical work, however, even if disguised and germane to the lecture topic, serve other, powerful roles in the teacher's professional work.

First, vignettes provide the teacher with opportunities to master conflict. Such mastery involves the reassessment of clinical work in which the teacher talks aloud about events that created anxiety. For example, a teacher who suddenly brings up a clinical case in order to highlight a central lecture point selects this specific case from all other possible cases because, on one level, it embodies unique personal meaning in this instructional context. It can be argued that even cases deemed successful still have elements of unfinished business that the teacher continues to process in the service of mastery strivings.

Second, the specific nature of the case itself may also speak indirectly to the teacher's unconscious perceptions of the classroom. A teacher's disclosure about a recalcitrant client, or a decision to excerpt for discussion a vignette from the class readings that deals with a troubled family system, takes on different meaning when the teacher realizes after the fact that several students have not been attending class. The pertinence of this type of insight speaks volumes about the impact of the teacher's unconscious perception on spontaneous disclosures about clinical cases. Here the teacher is not only selecting a case on the basis of its didactic merit, but also because it captures a critical aspect of the classroom environment about which the teacher is conflicted. It may even be suggested that at times the teacher unconsciously moves the lecture content in a certain direction in order to create a context for discussing a case that needs additional attention. Through this type of creative work, the teacher is able to impart knowledge to the class and continue to work over parts of his or her own casework and life contexts in which residual sentiment still lingers.

A teacher had prepared a lecture on the clinical features of paranoid pathology. At the start of the class, the teacher encouraged students to ask questions about the assigned readings. To no one's surprise, several students raised questions about an article with a clinical illustration involving a therapist's work with a paranoid patient. While students voiced concerns over what they

246 Training and Teaching the Mental Health Professional

perceived to be the confrontational nature of the therapist, the teacher began to formulate a general response. One student in particular appeared to be highly critical of the therapist's approach, and the teacher directed the response to that student.

The teacher advocated a less directive approach to therapy and in this regard was empathic with the tenor of student questioning surrounding the therapist's confrontational style with the paranoid client. The teacher, however, also noted that in some cases there may be justification for confrontation. This response did not sit well with the student toward whom the teacher had directed the response. The student felt strongly that the client in the case illustration was unsettled by the therapist's confrontational stance. A brief follow-up discussion ensued about the pros and cons of confronting clients, after which the teacher moved into the lecture material.

The presentation of lecture information was fairly cut and dried, save for one instance in which the teacher's train of thought was disrupted momentarily. This lapse occurred when the teacher was describing a personal experience in treating a stubborn, defiant client with paranoid trends. The teacher began to digress into a discussion of the types of difficulty encountered when treating highly defensive clients in general, but felt a brief clouding of consciousness during which the teacher forgot what had triggered this digression. Although slightly self-conscious about the way that this lapse might be perceived by the class, the teacher was able to quickly get back on track and returned to the lecture material after noting aloud, "Right, I was telling you about the client's defensiveness, and then I got sidetracked into talking about highly defended clients in general."

The teacher's focus then shifted from paranoid character pathology to an understanding of the paranoid process on a continuum that ranged from normal suspicion to severely delusional states. The purpose of this part of the lecture was to help students deepen their understanding of the fact that the types of suspicion that most people experience differ only in intensity from the experiences of more seriously disturbed individuals. Students appeared to grasp this point easily. As the class moved toward closure, a few questions were raised about an upcoming test. Because it was not unusual for students to ask about tests, the teacher did not give second thought to the underlying intent of the questions. As more questions were asked, however, it became apparent to the teacher that students were unusually anxious. Students wanted to know whether the teacher would be picayune about the types of questions asked and about grading criteria. One student wondered whether the teacher would develop "one of those impossible multiple-choice tests." Another student insisted that the teacher state exactly what would be on the test. There was also a request for the exact grading criteria that would be used, even before the teacher had a chance to state that the test had yet to be constructed.

The teacher felt somewhat cornered by the intensity of questioning and stated in a half-joking, half-serious tone, "Stop being so paranoid! It'll be fair." This comment was followed by some anxious laughter among the students, which triggered a twinge of guilt in the teacher, who then apologized playfully by remarking that the type of material presented in class "probably put all of us a bit on edge."

Grasping the dynamic that was salient in the here and now of the classroom experience, the teacher tried to help students understand that both teacher and students had unconsciously used the material presented in class to create a real learning moment for all involved. The teacher then offered as an explanation the idea that the lecture material dealing with paranoid pathology and suspicion may have actually sensitized students to anxieties associated with being deceived. It was suggested that the manifestation of this anxiety was evidenced by the rather anxious questioning of the teacher's intent with regard to the examination. Student suspicions had been incorporated into the classroom process in a way that articulated the very lecture point that the teacher had been presenting.

A review of this vignette draws together several ideas about psychoanalytic thinking that have been developed in this chapter in relation to classroom lecturing. Clearly, the lecture represents more than just the delivery of material to passive recipients. Instead, it is a dynamic process that has unconscious implications for student and teacher. For example, the teacher's momentary lapse of thought was probably triggered by unconscious associations to the client about whom the teacher had been talking right before digressing into a general discussion of highly defended clients. It may even be argued that the teacher's focus on one particular student's challenge to the readings also reflected a reenactment of a difficult therapy case; the student was unconsciously perceived as the obstinate client and contributed to the teacher's brief regression when presenting the lecture. The teacher's remark to students concerning their paranoia about an upcoming test and the subsequent apology may be understood in light of lecture content that had sensitized teacher and students to the dynamics of suspicion underscoring paranoid pathology. The teacher's empathy for the meaning of this material to students made it possible to demonstrate the experiential continuum that had been described as part of the lecture itself.

CHAPTER 10

Evaluation

Evaluation is another task for the teacher that can be understood within a psychoanalytic paradigm. The process of developing evaluation measures and grading student performance embraces many different psychoanalytic constructs, including transference, countertransference, and projective identification. For example, students may overemphasize in their test preparation a content area that they fantasize is more important to the teacher than other areas, use words when writing papers that they fantasize will curry the teacher's favor, and retaliate against what they feel is the teacher's subjectivity in grading when completing teacher evaluation forms anonymously. On the other side of the coin, teachers may experience miniepisodes of super-ego crises as they wrestle with fine discriminations in grading criteria, unwittingly act out against students by including poorly worded items on tests, and depersonalize the meaning of grades by offering minimal feedback on clinical papers in which students have invested great amounts of time and energy.

Four dimensions of the evaluation process can be understood from a psychoanalytic perspective: (1) dynamic considerations in test taking; (2) test format as a psychoanalytic analog; (3) dynamic considerations in grading students; and (4) student as instructor to the teacher. The first three of these areas address the role of the teacher as evaluator of the student. The fourth area addresses the evaluation process from a different angle by highlighting ways in which the student evaluates the teacher.

DYNAMIC CONSIDERATIONS IN TEST TAKING

The experience of taking tests, in class or in take-home form, modifies the routine tempo of classroom instruction and dialogue. Two areas in which modification in classroom structure during an evaluation affects underlying dynamics between teacher and student are the teacher's reduced interpersonal availability and dynamic features in the structure of evaluations.

The Teacher's Reduced Interpersonal Availability

The decrease in the teacher's direct support during an examination relative to the processes of lecturing and discussion represents an alteration in the teacher's interpersonal availability to students. Students who have grown accustomed to requesting and receiving clarification of questions on demand are now confronted with a teacher whose stance is distant. Students who would normally ask the teacher a question are now obliged to work on their own during an examination. Although such distance between teacher and student makes sense in light of the teacher's need to periodically evaluate student knowledge, it nevertheless represents a distinct change in the teacher's typical degree of support toward students.

Such modification in the teacher's usual style of relating to students has dynamic implications for the test-taking experience. During an evaluation period the teacher neither encourages collaboration among students nor has the freedom to answer questions with the same degree of directness as during lectures. This change in the teacher's response style represents a source of deprivation not only for students but also for the teacher. The teacher who derives gratification from being able to respond to student questions or from encouraging group discussion must now sit tight during what may be experienced as sink-or-swim time for students. In this respect, the evaluation context represents a psychological separation between teacher and student.

Although the evaluation is an encapsulated, time-limited separation that has been anticipated in conjunction with predetermined examination dates given in course syllabi, it still creates anxiety for student and teacher. Anxiety centers around display of competencies in which the self-esteem of students and teacher is affected by the outcome. Students who do well feel good about their skills; students who do not perform to expected levels may feel anxious, depressed, and angry. Teachers, too, may become buoyed or dispirited by the performances of students on evaluations. A student in whom the teacher has invested extra effort, but who does not perform to teacher expectation on an examination, may contribute to a teacher's sense of disappointment in himself or herself and in the student. In contrast, a teacher may feel affirmed by having contributed to the superior work of a student who demonstrates an astute grasp of course material. In some cases, the teacher may have indeed made a significant contribution to student performance, whereas in other cases, the teacher may inflate his or her contribution in order to maintain narcissistic equilibrium.

In reality, some students do well because of the teacher's ability to present material clearly. Here the teacher facilitates learning because of good teaching skill. In other situations, however, some students do well in spite of the teacher's limitations as an instructor. In this situation, students forge their own learning as a way of compensating for what they perceive to be the teacher's limitations as an instructor. In all cases, the separation between teacher and student that is one hallmark of taking tests is a forum for student competency to emerge and for the teacher to evaluate his or her contribution to the student's development.

The separation between teacher and student during an evaluation highlights the power differential in their roles. Students who hardly give thought to the teacher between classes may now find themselves fantasizing about the teacher with much greater frequency as they study class notes or prepare a paper in accord with the teacher's expectations. Images of the teacher lecturing to the class and responding to student questions mediate the student's relationship to the study material. Students may selectively recall classroom incidents in which fantasies of the teacher's power as grader were salient. For example, students may elaborate the meaning of one of the teacher's digressions in the middle of a lecture topic in an effort to determine whether the teacher was actually hinting at material that would be emphasized on the examination. Some other examples of student vulnerability in relation to perceptions of the teacher's power as grader may be evidenced by a student's asking the teacher whether the syllabus's omission of the usually stipulated double spacing for a paper in fact means that single spacing is permissible or pressing the teacher for specifics about which parts of a particular article assigned for class will be covered on a test.

These types of questions sensitize the teacher to student anxiety about grading and the need for grading accountability. But because these finely tuned questions also contrast with the more open-ended discussions that may have defined the class atmosphere during lecture presentations, the teacher may feel uncharacteristically cornered in the service of assuaging test anxiety in students. Moreover, the implicit psychological assumptions that are constant in the structure of an evaluation itself are also likely to arouse certain student sensitivities that contribute to the ways in which the class members react to the evaluation process.

Dynamic Features in the Structure of Evaluations

There are a series of explicit psychological assumptions placed on students by the teacher during an evaluation. Included among these assumptions are that the student will study, prepare, and work up to potential. It is reasonable for the teacher to assume that students who have paid hefty tuition in order to secure professional training are committed to their area of study and will therefore invest the necessary psychological resources in putting their best foot forward. Barring an unusual set of circumstances, this level of investment is quite likely to be the case. Indeed, these expectancies are often part of an ongoing dialogue in which the teacher encourages student inquisitiveness, seriousness, effort, and commitment to a chosen field of study.

There are, however, several implicit psychological assumptions that in many respects structure the psychology of the evaluation process for students. Included among the implicit assumptions of an evaluation are its submissive, dependent, exhibitionistic, and competitive features. These are clinical features that have much in common with the demands of test taking imposed on the client in the Rorschach situation as outlined by Schafer (1954).

Because of their implicit nature and relationship to unconscious processes, these assumptions are also less likely to be discussed openly as part of the psychology of being evaluated. Instead, they meld into the fabric of the evaluation process and are therefore less accessible to conscious awareness and not as easily defined as are explicit assumptions. Yet their inferred presence engages different characterological sensitivities in a way that makes even the most structured classroom examination a clinical activity. In moderation, each such feature may contribute to the student's ability to handle the pressures of being evaluated continually during a program of study. In extreme doses, however, each feature can work against the student's being able to approach the examination as a learning task.

Submissive Features

One of the defining attributes of an examination is that it requires students to submit to authority. Embedded within this assumption is the notion that students will do what they are told or risk consequence. Here submission to authority means that students are judged on the basis of their responses to measures that are devised and graded by the teacher. Furthermore, their responses must display some degree of conformity to what the teacher expects, even when teacher expectations are adumbrated rather than specified. Rarely, if ever, do students have the latitude to write their own test questions and grade their own answers in accord with their own sense of right and wrong. Instead, they prepare for a test with some general guidelines about examination content over which the teacher has ultimate authority.

From this perspective, it is understandable that students approach an examination by organizing their study around what the teacher is likely to find acceptable and unacceptable. Students who feel comfortable with the teacher's authority under these circumstances are able to prepare for a test or write a paper in the relative absence of conflictual thoughts or feelings about the nature of the task itself. Teachers who give students a voice in determining their destiny can assuage student fantasies of the teacher's rigidly authoritative stance around examinations. Student collaboration can be encouraged by providing reasonable rationales for testing format and content, remaining sensitive to what it means for a student to be tested or to have a paper reviewed, encouraging student involvement in developing examination content, and giving students individualized attention in response to their questions about grading decisions. In contrast, the teacher's insensitivity to the submissive quality of evaluations can leave some students feeling frustrated by the controlling nature of evaluations and by the sense that their frustrations will go unnoticed.

Dependent Features

The ability to relinquish control requires a capacity for depending on the benign intent of authority. Being able to trust those in positions of control makes it easier to make mistakes, be creative, and take risks without fearing punitive retribution. In this regard, the experience of submitting to a classroom evaluation requires not only compliance with authority, but also dependency on the fairness of those individuals in positions of control. The regressive nature of being evaluated implies a relinquishing of control and a trust in the ability of the teacher to build fairness and appropriate levels of challenge into the evaluation process. Students who are able to depend on the teacher to develop fair evaluations and grading criteria can approach the process of being evaluated in the belief that they will be assessed on their ability rather than on criteria that may otherwise be perceived as being inconsistent with expectation. Students who have difficulty trusting the teacher because of experiences in which either the present teacher or a past teacher misused authority are less likely to feel that the teacher's intent when structuring an evaluation measure is truly benign and in the service of enhancing their overall learning base.

Exhibitionistic Features

Another clinical feature of evaluations is that they provide students with a chance to parade their talents in front of the teacher. When taking a test or handing in a paper, the student is on center stage. The special circumstances surrounding an evaluation draw out sensitivities associated with having one's talents observed and judged. An evaluation is in many ways "show time" for students. For example, an evaluation mandating that the student express his or her skill in a format chosen by the teacher can stir fantasies associated with the student's need for affirmation. Students whose ideals are realistic can take pride in successful efforts without the intrusion of grandiose fantasies and can also handle the mild self-esteem fluctuations that accompany a less than perfect performance without hitting the depths of disappointment. At extremes, however, student fantasies can include the expectation of being either singled out because of exceptional talent or devalued because of insufficient competency. Attendant to these fantasies is the sense of depletion or futility that accompanies the failure to meet an ideal. Teachers who remain attuned to the narcissistic vulnerabilities engendered by evaluations are in a better position to respond empathically to student anxiety about being evaluated. In contrast, a dispassionate stance toward this same issue may serve only to deny the meanings engendered by the demand that students perform for the teacher as part of being evaluated.

Competitive Features

In addition to the submissive, dependent, and exhibitionistic aspects of the evaluation process, there is also a competitive element that is built into each and every evaluation. Students are eager to receive the teacher's affirmation based upon the quality of their work, but must perform under the pressure of knowing that the teacher will be assessing their performance in relation to other students. Although many students define their competitive efforts against their own standards, it is difficult to escape the reality that students often compete against each other for grades based on standards set by the teacher. In academic settings, competition for grades is fierce; differences in grade point averages among students, for example, can make a difference in awards of scholarship monies, strength of recommendation letters, and perceptions of suitability for different levels of training.

Because of the reward system set up around grades, competitive fantasies become roused along a continuum anchored by extremes of viewing the evaluation as do-or-die time or as a tension-packed situation from which retreat and underachievement are the most viable reactions. The teacher can mollify the competitive nature of evaluations by encouraging a classroom atmosphere in which students are invited to participate and share questions and answers. Here, students work together to find solutions to dilemmas posed by the teacher during the course of lectures, dilemmas posed by case presentations or readings.

TEST FORMAT AS PSYCHOANALYTIC ANALOG

The test format used by a teacher to evaluate students is a matter of individual preference and reality constraints. Teachers can choose from many different test formats when making decisions about how to best evaluate their-students: short answer, multiple choice, true-false, matching, compare-contrast essay, and case application are but some of the formats available to teachers. In addition, tests can be given in class or in take-home form. Factors influencing a teacher's test format include the type of content domain that is being tested and the amount of time available to administer and grade tests.

In addition to these considerations, the teacher may be confronted with another challenge when constructing a test format: Is it possible to make the examination a clinical task that fosters the integration of course material with the student's experience? Clearly, some courses lend themselves more readily to this type of test format than do other courses. For instance, it may be easier to integrate clinical case material into a course on child therapy than into one on psychometrics. In those courses that do have a more definite clinical focus, however, how can the teacher make the testing of course content a clinically meaningful activity within the context of the traditional classroom setting?

In order to begin to work toward developing an examination that speaks to these issues the teacher may ask her- or himself questions whose answers lend an apparent psychoanalytic focus to the examination format. For example, is it possible to construct a process-oriented test or to prepare a test that has sufficient structure to allow for some degree of standardization, but enough open terrain to allow the student's individuality to emerge? Is it possible to engage a student's unconscious in the test-taking process or to create a test format that encourages the student's identification with a client and a therapist? Is it possible to create test questions that allow the student to work creatively with clinical material or to involve students in the construction of the test itself so that they feel some control over the material that embodies the very concepts that they must articulate for a grade?

FIRST EXAMINATION

Background

Students taking an introductory course in psychoanalytic theory and therapy were presented with the following hypothetical clinical situation in a take-home examination format and were asked to limit their answers to a few questions to three typed pages. Students were required to work alone on the examination and were asked to direct any questions about the material to the teacher during office hours.

Clinical Material

Presenting Complaints

The client is a 31-year-old male, self-referred because of anxiety, angry outbursts toward his wife, parents, and 3-year-old daughter, periodic sleep problems, an extramarital affair, and chronic dissatisfaction with his work as a computer technician.

History of Complaints

The client, an only child, grew up in a dysfunctional family. Both parents had serious problems within their own families of origin, including histories of antisocial behavior for the paternal grandfather and chronic depression for the maternal grandmother. The client's parents fought with each other regularly, and the client has recollections of having grown up with a "knot" in his stomach. Although both parents gave the client attention and affection, they were sporadic in these regards. For example, the client recalled that when he was 8 years old he and a friend spent an entire day raking the family lawn with the client's father. The client recalled having what he felt was a "great day with dad." He was, therefore, quite devastated when his father remarked to his mother that their son seemed physically weaker than his friend. The client's mother was very critical of him and always seemed to be commenting on what the client was doing wrong. Her criticisms were confusing to the client because his mother was also the type of person in whom he could confide. She actually seemed drawn to her son as a confidant. Thus, when she criticized him, it really threw him for a loop because if he couldn't trust her, whom could he trust?

As a family, they rarely did things together. Indeed, the client's most prominent memories of his family were evening fights. Each night, the client's mother and father both would have cocktails, and an argument would almost invariably ensue. The client would usually go to his room in order to get some distance, but he would have great difficulty concentrating on his homework. He also had problems falling asleep. Both problems persist into adulthood.

The client recalls that a camp counselor was a positive role model. He recalled an instance of being at a sleepaway camp and having become quite upset when his parents got into a big argument during a parent visitation day. The client had been excited about their visiting and was very distressed and embarrassed by their arguing. In particular, he was upset to see his father "lose it." He recalled that his counselor was very understanding and explained to him that sometimes parents don't get along very well and that he understood how a kid could feel really bad, depressed, and confused about his parents' constant fighting. The counselor then spent some time with the client playing soccer and eating ice cream.

The client was a good student. He became interested in computers at an early age and eventually got a degree in this area. He met his wife at work; they dated for two years and then married. This was the first time that the client had been involved in a serious relationship. The client's wife came from a family in which she, too, had been the object of relentless criticism by her mother. The client was drawn to her in part because of his perception that they had something in common with regard to family of origin. Soon after marrying, however, the client found himself snapping at her in a highly critical tone. His wife told him early on that he was overreacting to her. "I'm not your mother!" she would say whenever the client made her feel inadequate.

The client's criticisms intensified after their daughter was born. It seemed as though the client's wife could do nothing right. It appeared, too, that the client would pick fights with her after talking about how unhappy he was at work. He felt that his job description was limiting, that there was little room for growth, and that he had made a wrong decision to work in computers. He was also quite angry with what he perceived as his wife's criticisms of their daughter, which drove the client "crazy." He was not sure what to do with himself, and he wondered aloud about pursuing an alternative vocational direction. This type of talk unsettled his wife, who was at first supportive of his wanting to go in other directions, but who soon grew uncomfortable with his chronic unhappiness at work and at home.

A few months prior to beginning therapy the client began an affair with a co-worker. He was lonely, felt depressed, and needed companionship; these were his stated reasons for the affair. He felt miserable, however, when he came home and looked at his young daughter.

He would say to himself, "What am I doing to my life?" It was at this point that he contacted a therapist for help.

Conditions of Therapy

The client was seen in weekly therapy by a male therapist whom the client had contacted after hearing him on a local talk-radio show. The therapist, who described himself as "a psychodynamic therapist," had been speaking about the reason that men have extramarital affairs (because they are really afraid of involvement with their own mothers).

For some reason, the client felt that this therapist could help him. He called the phone number that the therapist had given over the radio and spoke briefly to the therapist's answering service. The therapist then called the client back, and they set up an appointment. They met in the therapist's spacious home office on the same day and at the same time each week. Sessions would occasionally run well over the allotted time period, however, when the therapist felt that the client needed some extra support. The therapist would add this extra time to the client's fee by prorating the fee upwards. Seating was face to face. The therapist always poured the client coffee at the start of the session and insisted that the client address him by his first name. This informality made the client feel comfortable. The client paid the fee directly (no third-party payment) at the start of a new month for the period covering the prior month's sessions.

The client had had eight sessions when, arriving for his ninth session, he encountered the therapist's wife. They chatted briefly. She was an attractive woman and the client felt that they had made a "connection."

At the start of the ninth session, the client briefly mentioned that he had met the therapist's wife, who seemed nice. He then paused. Following the pause, he voiced disappointment in his progress. He claimed that he had made no demonstrable progress around the presenting problems and was having great difficulty in breaking off the extramarital affair. It depressed him, made him feel guilty, and led him to think of ending therapy. Indeed, he was afraid that he was on the verge of having another affair. He then told the therapist about a television show in which the person in charge issued a memo to staff stating that any employees who become romantically involved could not work on the same project. He then recalled another show in which a man's sense of failure led him to have an affair. All of this was disappointing to the client, and he labeled himself a failure.

The therapist encouraged him to be patient, stating, "Rome wasn't built in a day. You need to work some stuff out. Things will change, but you really can't push it." The client responded to this remark by saying, "I guess you're right. But I'm not sure what to do. I've been having thoughts of calling this telephone listing. It's the kind where you get to speak with women on the phone. I'm really freaked out. I know I won't do it, but just the thought scares the crap out of me. I have a young daughter! What does this say about me. Am I some kind of pervert? They should take all this stuff off the airwaves!"

The therapist reacted by telling the client that he was clearly projecting his own fear of being out of control onto other people, including the therapist, who had a radio show. The therapist felt that the client was actually becoming more at ease in therapy, that he really wanted to open up more and talk about deeper material, but that he was getting anxious about doing this. Calling the phone number to talk with women would be a sign of acting out.

The client responded by stating, "I'm not sure I buy that. I don't really see this as being related to your radio show." (The therapist thought to himself, "This is an example of transference resistance.")

The client then made manifest reference to the women who take phone calls and said, "I guess some people will do or say anything for a buck! The woman I'm having the affair with is a sweet-talker. Reminds me of my mother, in a way. It makes me uncomfortable because I've shared a lot with her, and I wonder in the back of my mind if this will come back to haunt me. I guess I need to think hard about ending that affair and not starting another one. I'll need your support to do this. It would be easier if we didn't have those open offices at work, you know, the kind where people have contact with each other all day long. It really does very little to promote a good work ethic." At this point the session came to an end.

Questions

1. How may the selfobject concept explain the client's reaction to his father and to his camp counselor during parent visitation day?
2. How may the concept of oedipal conflict help to explain the client's fantasy that he had made a "connection" with the therapist's wife?
3. How do you understand the concept of transference resistance in relation to the client's reaction to the therapist's interpretation about the meaning of making phone calls?
4. Identify deviant frame conditions.
5. First, explain how a communicative therapist would understand the meaning of the client's associations to the therapist's interpretation. Second, develop your understanding of the client's material into an interpretation.

SECOND EXAMINATION

Background

The same students who took the previous examination were given these instructions for their second examination.

Part 1

Please develop a vignette similar in format to the one that I developed for your first exam. Your vignette should include reason for referral, background, conditions of treatment, and clinical material. You should include sufficient background material to answer a question pertaining to the formation of the client's problems and sufficient clinical material to develop interpretations from the communicative, traditional, totalistic, and self psychological perspectives of analytic treatment.

There is a three-page limit to Part 1.

Part 2

Using material from the vignette, developed in Part 1, answer these questions. The limit is three pages, typed.

1. Integrate the concepts of the selfobject, ego functions, and drives in a way that helps to explain your client's problems.
2. Write a paper discussing how a communicative and either a totalistic, traditional, or self psychological therapist would develop an interpretation from the session material. Write the paper as if the therapist were saying it to the client.
3. Then analyze the structure of the interpretations. How are they alike? Different?

4. Take one of the three therapy approaches mentioned in Question 2, not including the classical model, and discuss how someone who adheres to that approach may understand Dora's decision to terminate treatment with Freud.

DISCUSSION

These two examinations are presented in detail in order to illustrate the ways that test construction can address important course concepts through a format that is sensitive to psychoanalytic processes. In the first examination, students were given an extensive case history and asked to integrate clinical material with course concepts. The take-home format gave students an opportunity to work at their own pace in a way that attempts to impose analog similarity to the analytic situation, but with the understanding that all work would be due on the same date.

By setting up this type of time frame, students have freedom to reflect on the examination material and entertain alternative answers before committing to a final response by a specified deadline date. The internal dialogues that students set up in developing their answers also bring them in touch with different types of thoughts and feelings about themselves, the course, and the teacher as one way of deriving new insights about the meaning of the clinical material. For example, some students may reach new personal understanding by integrating course concepts with events from their own histories, which they recollect in connection with reviewing the present case material. They may access new insights into their own work as clinicians as a byproduct of the intensity with which they assess the dynamics between client and therapist in the session. They may find themselves preoccupied with fantasies about the teacher as they work on the examination. Such fantasies may help students deepen their appreciation for transference and countertransference and provide a readily accessible experience base from which to augment their understanding of the examination material.

The second examination represents a continuation of the process that started with the first examination, but with slight modifications. Here students were asked to create their own hypothetical clinical material, using as a model the case material that had been developed by the teacher for the first examination. By inviting students to prepare the clinical material, the teacher also sought to nurture the integration of their unconscious creativity. In addition, students were given more control over the grading process by virtue of increased responsibility for the quality of clinical material in relation to the questions to which they would have to respond. Students were also given increased control over their grade, which would be dependent on their ability to work with their own material rather than adjust to the material developed by the teacher. As such, the examination gave them room to deliberate, engage, and articulate their own conceptions of a clinical experience grounded in fundamental concepts within the course content domain.

DYNAMIC CONSIDERATIONS IN GRADING STUDENTS

Classroom Learning

Tests and Papers

Intimately related to the format of evaluation is the development of criteria for grading. The teacher must make decisions about how many evaluation measures to include during a course and when to give them, how to weight them in the overall grading scheme, and how to justify different grading systems to students. Each decision evolves from dynamic processes that bear the stamp of the individual teacher.

Tests offering students dichotomous choices all but eliminate shadings from the teacher's grading decisions. In these cases, an answer is either right or wrong, with point distribution meted according to accuracy in an all-or-nothing format. Such tests can be graded by hand or computer; they minimize the teacher's emotional involvement in grading, save for decisions about curving skewed grade distributions. The advantages of this type of evaluation are that it brings efficiency to the evaluation process and it is suited to certain types of courses within the mental health curriculum.

In contrast to forced-choice evaluations, there are several other evaluation formats that impose different psychological demands on the teacher. Essay tests, application tests involving the type of clinical reasoning suggested in the previous section, and clinical papers are three such evaluation measures that introduce more subjectivity into the grading process than do forced-choice tests. When grading essays, applications, and papers, the teacher must discriminate answers along a point continuum that is both reasonable and defensible. Indeed, it should not surprise the teacher whose grading involves subjectivity that students request justification of the teacher's point system when they notice slight discrepancies between points lost on their answer relative to what they perceive as a comparable answer of a peer. Similar concerns may arise for students who are asked to write clinical papers. Because paper topics often reflect areas that are particularly meaningful to students, it may be especially difficult for a student to understand the teacher's rationale for a grade that falls below the student's expectation.

Using broad grading criteria when evaluating essays or papers affords the teacher latitude when making grade decisions that minimize hair splitting in favor of reading and critiquing the student's work in a broad context.

The development of a grading system is itself a reflection of the teacher's personal taste. How does a teacher decide to take off five points for one answer and three points for another answer? Are decisions made on a purely rational basis before reviewing any answers or after reviewing every answer once before even attempting to mark a paper? Or does the teacher first read the answers of outstanding students and then use the quality of these answers as a baseline against which to evaluate all other answers? Is there a risk of bias if this system is adopted? These are but some of the questions that emerge in response to the psychological challenge of grading students.

In attempting to answer these questions, the teacher with psychoanalytic interests is invariably sensitized to the way in which the process of grading can be understood from a psychoanalytic perspective. The superego rustlings that can either interfere with or enhance the grading process represent one example of how the teacher's sense of fair play can become entangled with fantasies of hurting people as well as with the undoing efforts that help keep these feelings in check. Similarly, the wish to support a student in whom the teacher has a vested interest, but whose test performance does not warrant a top grade, can also be a setting in which the teacher's conscientiousness works overtime in order to assuage anxiety associated with a grading decision.

Most telling in the grading process is the teacher's own conscious and unconscious identifications with the meaning of grades. Grading students brings the teacher in contact with his or her own history as a student. The grading process leads the teacher to reflect upon what it means to be graded, to receive grades, and to share grades with classmates. The teacher may recall feeling elated when achieving and depressed when grades did not meet self or other expectations. A teacher who struggled with a particular course as a student may, in an extreme situation, hesitate to teach a similar course many years later. At the other extreme, the teacher may agree to teach the course, but protect against reliving the stress felt when taking that same course as a student by either unwittingly inflating grades or instituting a rigorous grading process that makes the attainment of high marks nearly impossible.

Identifications with certain students may touch the teacher in a personal way. When grading, the teacher strives to balance his or her own identification with students against a responsive grading system in which the teacher strives for fairness in the service of helping students identify strengths and weaknesses. Yet there are times when students take umbrage with their grades and challenge the teacher to clarify his or her grading criteria. In such cases, the teacher offers feedback in the form of a clinical intervention. By attempting to respond to student concerns empathically, the teacher displays appreciation for the destabilizing effect of low grades on self-esteem, offers recommendations for remediation, and remains open to modifying the grade if warranted.

When the teacher feels that a student's grade warrants change, then other students who meet the revised grading criteria on a specific item or on several questions should also be informed of the new criteria. Changes in grades under these conditions can be handled by inviting students whose answers meet the new criteria to present their work to the teacher for grade revision. The teacher's willingness to acknowledge justifiable oversights in grading decisions at the behest of student input can create an ambience in which students experience the teacher as being open and accepting. Thus students take away an empathic introject rather than the feeling of dismissal. Even in situations in which grade modification does not appear to be warranted, the teacher can remain empathic and encourage student self-expression while still holding firm to the original grading decision.

STUDENT AS INSTRUCTOR TO THE TEACHER

For the psychoanalytic educator, the profession of teaching provides endless opportunities to engage in psychoanalytic dialogue. Through preparation, lecturing, and evaluating, the teacher always has available a rich lode of interpersonal data from which to refine his or her understanding of psychoanalytic theory in relation to instructional processes. As a clinical entity, psychoanalytic theory is centered on the mutuality of influence that shapes the relationship between therapist and client. In psychoanalytic therapy, the client impacts the therapist, but the therapist also impacts the client.

One of the ways in which psychoanalytic theory informs the instructional process is through the notion that, in addition to being an instructor to the student, the teacher is also instructed by the student. The teacher learns from his or her students in many ways—by being mindful of the role that the classroom framework plays in providing a measure of hold and stability to the instructional process, by processing private reactions to students, by trying to understand the different reactions that students have to their teacher, and by using student questions to develop a comprehensive understanding of course material.

End-of-course evaluations are a very real learning instrument for the teacher. Positive feedback can be affirming, but the teacher must also be able to hear about areas that need attention. For example, student concerns about the teacher's receptiveness to questions, attitude when challenged, and openness to alternative viewpoints can assist the teacher in taking the steps needed in order to make the classroom setting a safe place for students. Some other areas of the teacher's performance to which students may be sensitive include the promptness with which tests and papers are returned, the quality of photocopying for articles that were placed on reserve, and the level of sophistication of the course relative to student expectations. Because the teacher's self-esteem is vulnerable to the evaluation process, there is a need to keep in perspective the meaning of student comments that seem to aggrandize or attack the teacher's competency. The teacher's ability to synthesize and utilize student feedback serves ultimately to make the classroom a safe learning environment for all concerned.

REFERENCES

Adelson, M. J. (1995). Clinical supervision of therapists with difficult-to-treat patients. *Bulletin of the Menninger Clinic* 59:32–52.

Adler, G. (1972). Helplessness in the helper. *British Journal of Medical Psychology* 45:315–326.

Adler, G., and Rhine, M. W. (1988). The selfobject function of projective identification. *Bulletin of the Menninger Clinic* 52:473–491.

Allen, D. W. (1967). Exhibitionistic and voyeuristic conflicts in learning and functioning. *Psychoanalytic Quarterly* 36:546–570.

Allison, J., Blatt, S. J., and Zimet, C. Z. (1968). *The Interpretation of Psychological Tests*. New York: Harper & Row.

Appelbaum, A. (1972). On hearing, presenting and discussing scientific papers. *Bulletin of the Menninger Clinic* 36:546–550.

Baker, H. S., and Baker, M. N. (1987). Heinz Kohut's self psychology: an overview. *American Journal of Psychiatry* 144:1–9.

Barbanel, L. (1994). Psychoanalysis and school psychology. *Psychoanalytic Psychology* 11:275–284.

Basch, M. F. (1989). The teacher, the transference, and development. In *Learning and Education: Psychoanalytic Perspectives*, ed. K. Field, B. J. Cohler, and G. Wool, pp. 771–787. Madison, CT: International Universities Press.

Bellak, L. (1975). *The T.A.T., C.A.T. and S.A.T. in Clinical Use*. New York: Grune & Stratton.

Bennett, B. E., Bryant, B. K., Vanden Bos, G. R., and Greenwood, A. (1990). *Professional Liability and Risk Management*. Washington, DC: American Psychological Association.

Berg, M. (1984). Expanding the parameters of psychological testing. *Bulletin of the Menninger Clinic* 48:10–24.

Bettelheim, B. (1950). *Love Is Not Enough*. New York: Collier Books.

_____ (1955). *Truants from Life*. New York: Free Press.

_____ (1974). *A Home for the Heart*. New York: Alfred Knopf.

_____ (1982). *Freud and Man's Soul*. New York: Vintage Books.

Brookfield, S. D. (1990). *The Skillful Teacher*. San Francisco, CA: Jossey-Bass.

Brown, R. S., Finkin, M. W., Levin, B., et al. (1994). Academic freedom and sexual harrassment. *Academe*, 80:64–72.

Bryant, K. N. (1964). Some clinical notes on reading disability: a case study. *Bulletin of the Menninger Clinic* 28:323–338.

Bullough, R. V., Jr., Knowles, J. G., and Crow, N. A. (1991). *Emerging as a Teacher.* New York: Routledge.

Burlingham, D. (1937). Problem of the psychoanalytic educator. *Zeitschrift für Psychoanalytische Pedagogik* 11:91–97.

Casement, P. (1985). *Learning from the Patient.* New York: Guilford.

Centra, J. A. (1993). *Reflective Faculty Evaluation: Enhancing Teaching and Determining Faculty Effectiveness.* San Francisco, CA: Jossey-Bass.

Cheifetz, L. G. (1984). Framework violations in psychotherapy with clinic patients. In *Listening and Interpreting: The Challenge of the Work of Robert Langs,* ed. J. Raney, pp. 215–254. New York: Jason Aronson.

Cohler, B. J. (1989). Psychoanalysis and education: motive, memory, and self. In *Learning and Education: Psychoanalytic Perspectives,* ed. K. Field, B. J. Cohler, and G. Wool, pp. 11–83. Madison, CT: International Universities Press.

Connors, M. E. (1994). Symptom formation: an integrative self psychological perspective. *Psychoanalytic Psychology* 11:509–523.

Cormier, L. S., and Bernard, J. M. (1982). Ethical and legal responsibilities of clinical supervisors. *The Personnel Guidance Journal* 60:486–491.

Cozzarelli, L. A., and Silin, M. (1989). The effects of narcissistic transferences on the teaching–learning process. In *Learning and Education: Psychoanalytic Perspectives,* ed. K. Field, B. J. Cohler, and G. Wool, pp. 809–823. Madison, CT: International Universities Press.

Crisp, P. (1986). Projective identification: an attempt at clarification. *Journal of the Melanie Klein Society* 4:47–76.

Cross, P. K. (1991). *Adults as Learners: Increasing Participation and Facilitating Learning.* San Francisco, CA: Jossey-Bass.

Davis, B. G. (1993). *Tools for Teaching.* San Francisco, CA: Jossey-Bass.

Dewald, P. A. (1987). *Learning Processes in Psychoanalytic Supervision: Complexities and Challenges.* Madison, CT: International Universities Press.

Diagnostic and Statistical Manual of Mental Disorders, 4th ed. (1994). Washington, DC: American Psychiatric Association.

Doehrman, M. J. G. (1976). Parallel processes in supervision and psychotherapy. *Bulletin of the Menninger Clinic* 40.

Ebel, K. E. (1988). *The Craft of Teaching.* San Francisco, CA:

Jossey-Bass.

Eber, M., and Kunz, L. B. (1984). The desire to help others. *Bulletin of the Menninger Clinic* 48:125–140.

Ekstein, R. (1964a). The boundary line between education and psychoanalysis. *Reiss-Davis Clinic Bulletin* 1:26–28.

———— (1964b). The learning process: from learning for love to love of learning. *Reiss-Davis Clinic Bulletin* 1:29–32.

Ekstein, R., and Motto, R. L. (1963). Psychoanalysis and education: a reappraisal. *Psychoanalytic Review* 51:29–44.

Ekstein, R., and Wallerstein, R. (1958). *The Teaching and Learning of Psychotherapy*. New York: International Universities Press.

Ellis, A., and Grieger, R., eds. (1977). *Handbook of Rational-Emotive Therapy*. New York: Springer.

Exner, J. E., Jr. (1993). *The Rorschach: A Comprehensive System*, vol. 1, 3rd ed. New York: Wiley.

Fairbairn, W. R. D. (1963). Synopsis of an object-relations theory of the personality. *International Journal of Psycho-Analysis* 44:224–225.

Field, K. (1989). Some reflections on the student–teacher dialogue: a psychoanalytic perspective. In *Learning and Education: Psychoanalytic Perspectives*, ed. K. Field, B. J. Cohler, and G. Wool, pp. 851–926. Madison, CT: International Universities Press.

Field, K., Cohler, B. J., and Wool, G., eds. (1989). *Learning and Education: Psychoanalytic Perspectives*. Madison, CT: International Universities Press.

Fitzgerald, L. F., and Osipow, S. H. (1986). An occupational analysis of counseling psychology: how special is the specialty? *American Psychologist* 41:535–541.

Freud, A. (1935/1979). *Psycho-analysis for Teachers and Parents*. New York: Norton.

Freud, S. (1905). Fragment of an analysis of a case of hysteria. *Standard Edition* 12:3–122.

———— (1912a). The dynamics of the transference. *Standard Edition* 12:97–108.

———— (1912b). Recommendations to physicians practising psycho-analysis. *Standard Edition* 12:109–120.

———— (1913). On beginning the treatment. *Standard Edition* 12:121–144.

———— (1914). Remembering, repeating and working through. *Standard Edition* 12:145–156.

———— (1915). Observations on transference love. *Standard Edi-

tion 12:157–171.

_____ (1925). Preface to Aichorn's *Wayward Youth*. *Standard Edition* 19:273–275.

Garber, B. (1989). Deficits in empathy in the learning disabled child. In *Learning and Education: Psychoanalytic Perspectives.* ed. K. Field, B. J. Cohler, and G. Wool, pp. 617–635. Madison, CT: International Universities Press.

Gardner, R. M. (1994). *On Trying to Teach*. Hillsdale, NJ: Analytic Press.

Gill, M. M. (1982). *Analysis of Transference. Volume I: Theory and Technique*. New York: International Universities Press.

Goldberg, C. (1986). *On Being a Psychotherapist: The Journey of the Healer*. New York: Gardner.

Goldsmith, B. L. (1994). Some thoughts on teaching trainees about transference: commentary on Kane, Tryon and Halligan. *Journal of College Student Psychotherapy* 8:29–34.

Greenberg, J. R., and Mitchell, J. A. (1983). *Object Relations in Psychoanalytic Theory*. Cambridge, MA: Harvard University Press.

Greer, J. M. (1994). "Return of the repressed" in the analysis of an adult incest survivor: a case study and some tentative generalizations. *Psychoanalytic Psychology* 11:545–561.

Groth-Marnat, G. (1990). *Handbook of Psychological Assessment*, 2nd ed. New York: Wiley.

Grotstein, J. S. (1986). *Splitting and Projective Identification*. Northvale, NJ: Jason Aronson.

Grumet, M. R. (1994). Reading the relations of teaching. *Psychoanalytic Psychology* 11:253–264.

Guy, J. D. (1987). *The Personal Life of the Psychotherapist*. New York: Wiley.

Harrar, W. R., VandeCreek, L., and Knapp, S. (1990). Ethical and legal aspects of clinical supervision. *Professional Psychology: Research and Practice* 21:37–41.

Harris, H. I. (1966). Drop-out and negative institutional transference. *American Journal of Psychotherapy* 20:664–668.

Hartmann, H. (1958). *Ego Psychology and the Problem of Adaptation*. New York: International Universities Press.

Jones, R. M. (1960). *An Application of Psychoanalysis to Education*. Springfield, IL: Charles C Thomas.

Kaley, H. (1993). Psychoanalysis and education: attitude and process. *Psychoanalytic Psychology* 10:93–103.

_____ (1994). Organizer's discussion. *Psychoanalytic Psychology* 11:285–290.

Kane, A. S., Tryon, G. S., and Halligan, F. R. (1994). A developmental framework for assisting trainees in a college counseling center in their use of transference and countertransference to conceptualize clients' problems. *Journal of College Student Psychotherapy* 8:5–22.

Kaye, S. (1994). The place of depression in dysfunctional learning. *Psychoanalytic Psychology* 11:265–274.

Keith-Spiegel, P., and Koocher, G. P. (1985). *Ethics in Psychology: Professional Standards and Cases*. New York: Random House.

Kernberg, O. (1975). *Borderline Conditions and Pathological Narcissism*. New York: Jason Aronson.

——— (1980). *Internal World and External Reality: Object Relations Theory Applied*. New York: Jason Aronson.

——— (1987). Projection and projective identification: developmental and clinical aspects. *Journal of the American Psychoanalytic Association* 35:795–819.

Kissen, M., ed. (1986). *Assessing Object Relations*. Madison, CT: International Universities Press.

Klein, E. (1949). Psychoanalytic aspects of school problems. *Psychoanalytic Study of the Child* 3–4: 369–390. New York: International Universities Press.

Klein, M. (1975). The early development of the conscious in the child. In *Melanie Klein: Love, Guilt and Reparation and Other Works 1921–1945*, pp. 248–257. New York: Free Press.

Kohut, H. (1971). *The Analysis of the Self*. New York: International Universities Press.

——— (1977). *The Restoration of the Self*. New York: International Universities Press.

Kolstoe, O. P. (1975). *College Professoring*. Carbondale and Evanston, IL: Southern Illinois University Press.

Koppitz, E. M. (1975). *The Bender Gestalt Test for Young Children: Volume II: Research and Application 1963–1973*. New York: Grune & Stratton.

Kris, E. (1948). On psychoanalysis and education. *American Journal of Orthopsychiatry* 18:622–635.

Kwawer, J. S., Lerner, H. D., Lerner, P. M., and Sugarman, A., eds. (1980). *Borderline Phenomena and the Rorschach Test*. New York: International Universities Press.

Lane, R. C., and Meisels, M., eds. (1994). *A History of the Division of Psychoanalysis of the American Psychological Association*. Hillsdale, NJ: Lawrence Erlbaum.

Langs, R. (1976a). *The Therapeutic Interaction: Volume I*. New York: Jason Aronson.

_____ (1976b). *The Therapeutic Interaction: Volume II*. New York: Jason Aronson.

_____ (1982a). *The Psychotherapeutic Conspiracy*. New York: Jason Aronson.

_____ (1982b). *Psychotherapy: A Basic Text*. New York: Jason Aronson.

_____ (1985). *Workbooks for Psychotherapists: Vol. III—Intervening and Validating*. Emerson, NJ: Newconcept Press.

_____ (1992a). The self-processing class and the psychotherapy frame. *American Journal of Psychotherapy* 1:75–90.

_____ (1992b). Boundaries and frames: non-transference in teaching. *International Journal of Communicative Psychoanalysis and Psychotherapy* 7:125–130.

_____ (1994). *Doing Supervision and Being Supervised*. London: Karnac.

Lerner, P. (1991). *Psychoanalytic Theory and the Rorschach*. Hillsdale, NJ: Analytic Press.

_____ (1994). Treatment issues in a case of possible multiple personality disorder. *Psychoanalytic Psychology* 11:563–574.

Liss, E. (1941). The failing student. *American Journal of Orthopsychiatry* 11:712–718.

Lubin, M. (1984–1985). Another source of danger for psychotherapists: the supervisory introject. *International Journal of Psycho-analytic Psychotherapy*, vol. 11, ed. R. Langs, pp. 25–45. New York: Jason Aronson.

Lubin, M., and Stricker, G. (1992). Teaching the core curriculum. In *The Core Curriculum in Professional Psychology*, ed. R. L. Peterson, J. D. McHolland, R. J. Bent, et al., pp. 43–47. Washington, DC: American Psychological Association and National Council of Schools of Professional Psychology.

Lunardi, P. M. (1993). *Communicative paradigms applied to role play in an educational setting*. Unpublished master's thesis, Immaculata College, Immaculata, PA.

Mahler, M. S., Pine, F., and Bergman, A. (1975). *The Psychological Birth of the Human Infant*. New York: Basic Books.

Maroda, K. (1994). *The Power of Countertransference*. Northvale, NJ: Jason Aronson.

Masson, J. M. (1984). *The Assault on the Truth: Freud's Suppression of the Seduction Theory*. New York: Penguin.

Mehlman, E., and Glickauf-Hughes, C. (1994). Understanding

developmental needs of college students in mentoring relationships with professors. *Journal of College Student Psychotherapy* 8:39–53.

Meisels, M., and Shapiro, E. R., eds. (1990). *Tradition and Innovation in Psychoanalytic Education: Clark Conference of Psychoanalytic Training of Psychologists.* Hillsdale, NJ: Lawrence Erlbaum.

Merriam, S. B., and Cafferella, R. S. (1991). *Learning in Adulthood.* San Francisco, CA: Jossey-Bass.

Mitchell, S. A. (1993). *Hope and Dread in Psychoanalysis.* New York: Basic Books.

Murray, H. A. (1938). *Explorations in Personality.* New York: Oxford University Press.

Murray, J. F. (1995). On objects, transference, and two-person psychology: a critique of the new seduction theory. *Psychoanalytic Psychology* 12:31–41.

Oberndorf, C. P. (1939). The feeling of stupidity. *International Journal of Psycho-Analysis* 20:443–451.

Ogden, T. H. (1979). On projective identification. *International Journal of Psycho-Analysis* 60:357–373.

Overholser, J. C., and Fine, M. A. (1990). Defining the boundaries of professional competence: managing subtle cases of clinical incompetence. *Professional Psychology: Research and Practice* 21:462–469.

Peller, L. E. (1956). The school's role in promoting sublimation. *Psychoanalytic Study of the Child* 2:437–449. New York: International Universities Press.

Pine, F. (1990). *Drive, Ego, Object and Self: A Synthesis for Clinical Work.* New York: Basic Books.

Pulver, S. E. (1993). The eclectic analyst: or the many roads to insight and change. *Journal of the American Psychoanalytic Association* 41:339–357.

Rapaport, D., Gill, M. M., and Schafer, R. (1968). *Diagnostic Psychological Testing*, ed. R. Holt. New York: International Universities Press.

Rodolfa, E., Hall, T., Davena, A., et al. (1994). The management of sexual feelings in therapy. *Professional Psychology: Research and Practice* 25:168–172.

Rowe, C. E., and Mac Isaac, D. S. (1989). *Empathic Attunement: The Technique of Self Psychology.* Northvale, NJ: Jason Aronson.

Rychlak, J. F. (1973). *Introduction to Personality and Psychotherapy: A Theory Construction Approach.* Boston, MA:

Houghton Mifflin.

Salzberger-Wittenberg, I., Henry, G., and Osborne, E. (1983). *The Emotional Experience of Learning and Teaching.* London: Routledge & Kegan Paul.

Schafer, R. (1948). *Clinical Application of Psychological Tests.* New York: International Universities Press.

———— (1954). *Psychoanalytic Interpretation in Rorschach Testing.* New York: Grune & Stratton.

———— (1967). *Projective Testing and Psychoanalysis.* New York: International Universities Press.

———— (1992). *Retelling a Life: Narration and Dialogue in Psychoanalysis.* New York: Basic Books.

Schwaber, E. A., ed. (1985). *The Transference in Psychotherapy: Clinical Management.* New York: International Universities Press.

Shapiro, D. (1965). *Neurotic Styles.* New York: Basic Books.

Shore, K. (1994). To stand up and say "No!" *Psychologist Psychoanalyst* 14:4–5.

Shulman, M. E. (1994). Managed care and health care reform: appreciating full threat. *Psychologist Psychoanalyst* 14:5–8.

Shur, R. (1994). *Countertransference Enactment.* Northvale, NJ: Jason Aronson.

Smith, D. L. (1991). *Hidden Conversations: An Introduction to Communicative Psychoanalysis.* London: Routledge.

Steenbarger, B. N. (1992). Intentionalizing brief college student psychotherapy. *Journal of College Student Psychotherapy* 7:47–61.

Stone, L. (1984). *Transference and Its Context.* Northvale, NJ: Jason Aronson.

Sugarman, A. (1981). Diagnostic use of countertransference reactions in psychological testing. *Bulletin of the Menninger Clinic* 45:473–490.

Sutherland, R. L. (1951). An application of the theory of psychosexual development to the learning process. *Bulletin of the Menninger Clinic* 15:91–99.

Tansey, M. J., and Burke, W. F. (1989). *Understanding Countertransference: From Projective Identification to Empathy.* Hillsdale, NJ: Analytic Press.

Thompson, R., and Appelbaum, D. (1995). Psychoanalysis and graduate school training: a survey of students' experiences. *Psychologist Psychoanalyst* 15:17–19.

Tipton, R. M., Watkins, C. E., Jr., and Ritz, S. (1991). Selection, training and career preparation of predoctoral interns in psychology. *Professional Psychology: Research and Practice* 22:60–67.

Trawinski, C. J. (1990). An analysis of shift in intervention style. *Bulletin of the Society for Psychoanalytic Psychotherapy* 5:5–19.

Troise, F. P. (1993). Freud's research understanding of transference: transference proper or role evocation. *International Journal of Communicative Psychoanalysis and Psychotherapy* 8:55–66.

Usher, R., and Edwards, R. (1994). *Postmodernism and Education*. London: Routledge.

Vlosky, M. (1984). Community mental health clients' rights and the therapeutic frame. In *Listening and Interpreting: The Challenge of the Work of Robert Langs*, ed. J. Raney, pp. 255–266. New York: Jason Aronson.

Watkins, C. E., Jr. (1985). Countertransference: its impact on the counseling situation. *Journal of Counseling and Development* 63:356–359.

Watkins, C. E., Jr., Schneider, L. J., Manus, M., and Hunton-Shoup, J. (1990). Terminal master's-level training in counseling psychology: skills, competencies and student interests. *Professional Psychology: Research and Practice* 21:216–218.

Weisberg, I. (1994). Brief, time-limited psychotherapy and the communicative approach. *The International Journal of Communicative Psychoanalysis and Psychotherapy* 8:105–108.

Winnicott, D. W. (1960). The theory of the parent–infant relationship. In *The Maturational Processes and the Facilitating Environment*, pp. 37–55. New York: International Universities Press.

——— (1986). *Holding and Interpretation: Fragment of an Analysis*. New York: Grove.

Wisocki, P. A., Grebstein, L. C., and Hunt, J. B. (1994). Directors of clinical training: an insider's perspective. *Professional Psychology: Research and Practice* 25:482–488.

Wolf, E. S. (1989). The psychoanalytic self psychologist looks at learning. In *Learning and Education: Psychoanalytic Perspectives*, ed. K. Field, B. J. Cohler, and G. Wool, pp. 377–393. Madison, CT: International Universities Press.

Wool, G. (1989). Relational aspects of learning: the learning alliance. In *Learning and Education: Psychoanalytic Perspectives*, ed. K. Field, B. J. Cohler, and G. Wool, pp.

733–770. Madison, CT: International Universities Press.

Yalof, J. (1991). Review of *Understanding Countertransference: From Projective Identification to Empathy* by M. J. Tansey and W. F. Burke. *Society for Psychoanalytic Psychotherapy Bulletin* 6:39–40.

_____ (1993). Some impressions of the phenomenology of the Rorschach student: a teacher's perspective. *Society for Personality Assessment Exchange* 3:11–12.

Zabarenko, L. M., and Zabarenko, R. N. (1974). Psychoanalytic contributions for a theory of instruction. *Annals of Psychoanalysis* 2:323–345.

CREDITS

The author gratefully acknowledges permission to quote from the following sources:

"On the Classroom Teaching of Psychoanalytic Theory and Therapy: A Teacher's Perspective," by Jed A. Yalof, in *International Journal of Communicative Psychoanalysis and Psychotherapy*, vol. 7(3–4): pp. 119–124. Copyright © 1992 by the *International Journal of Communicative Psychoanalysis and Psychotherapy*.

"Some Impressions of the Phenomenology of the Rorschach Student: A Teacher's Perspective," by Jed A. Yalof, in *Society for Personality Assessment Exchange*, vol. 3(2): pp. 11–12. Copyright © 1993 by the Society for Personality Assessment.

From *The Maturational Processes and the Facilitating Environment*, by D. W. Winnicott. Copyright © 1960 by International Universities Press.

From *Learning and Education: Psychoanalytic Perspectives*, edited by K. Field, B. J. Cohler, and G. Wool. Copyright a 1989 by International Universities Press.

INDEX

Abnormal behavior courses,
180–183
Absence from class
by students, 143–144
by teachers, 152–153
Academic institutions. *See
also* Classroom frame
clinical supervision in,
11–12
management of change in,
64–65
organizational dynamics in,
58–66, 104–106,
165–166
physical security in, 66–67
predictability in, 65–66,
104–106
professional identity
within, 29–30
psychoanalytic education
in, 9–12
role models in, 67–68
rules and expectations in,
61–62, 68–71, 89–90,
92

safe learning environment
in, 62–65, 64–65,
108–110, 224–225
salaries in, 85, 104–106
status of psychoanalytic
theory in, 9–11
structure in, 50–51, 59–61
supportive, 58–71,
104–106, 224–225
Academic problems. *See*
Inappropriate behavior;
Learning problems
Acting out. *See* Inappropriate
behavior
Active orality, 117–118, 127
Adler, G., 48
Adult learners, 44–45,
231–232
Aloof therapist, 187–188
Alternative classroom
frames, 11–12, 81–82,
231–232
Ambiguity tolerance, 40–42
American Psychological
Association, 7, 10

Analytic neutrality, 39–40,
     90, 139–140, 149–150.
     See also Teacher
     neutrality
Appelbaum, A., 10, 237–238
Attention-deficit disorder, 25
Authority conflicts, 45–46,
     118–119, 151–160,
     240–241, 258–261

Behavioral problems. *See*
     Inappropriate behavior
Bellak, L., 120
Benign countertransference,
     198–199
Bettelheim, B., 5, 116
Boundary management. *See*
     Classroom frame;
     Therapeutic frame
Brookfield, S. D., 78, 95, 231
Bryant, K. N., 25
Burke, W. F., 38, 161–162
Burlingham, D., 14
Burnout
     in teachers, 50–51
     in therapists, 47–50

Caretaker role, 19–23, 56–58,
     121–124
Case presentations. *See*
     Clinical seminars
Casement, P., 25
Centra, J. A., 231
Character styles, 216–221
Cheifetz, L. G., 193
Childhood depression, 25
Childhood development, 14,
     18–23, 57–58, 115–117.
     See also Learning

Childhood education, 13–14
Classroom dynamics. *See also*
     Classroom frame;
     Learning
clinical material affects,
     90–92, 174–184,
     193–202, 244–249
countertransference in,
     148–167, 197–200,
     240–242
ego psychology and, 120,
     127–128
during evaluation, 254–261
extrainstructional contacts
     and, 100–102,
     145–146, 156–157
grading and, 92–93,
     154–156, 253–254,
     272–275
idealization of teachers
     and, 16, 21–22,
     175–176
interpersonal processes in,
     135–138, 140–148,
     150–167, 197–200,
     240–242
intrapsychic processes in,
     16–26, 113–125,
     127–132
during lectures, 231–249
object relations and, 121,
     128–129
projective identification in,
     160–167
psychoanalytic therapy
     contrasted to, 233–236
psychosexuality and,
     18–19, 117–119, 127,
     131–132

self psychology and,
 122–124, 129–130
self-disclosure and, 90–93,
 126–127, 201,
 244–249
teacher intervention in,
 130–132, 147–148,
 236–237
transference in, 16, 20,
 140–148, 160–167
Classroom frame, 81–110. *See
 also* Academic
 institutions; Classroom
 dynamics; Therapeutic
 frame
breaks in, 83–84, 141–148,
 150–160, 162–165
in clinical seminars,
 193–202
concept of, 81–83
confidentiality in, 82,
 85–86, 106–108
course evaluation in, 86,
 108–110
course syllabi in, 84,
 89–90
during evaluation, 254–271
extrainstructional contact
 in, 85, 100–102
feedback in, 84–85, 93–98
fees in, 82, 85, 104–106
grading criteria in,
 154–156, 271–275
interventions, 158–160,
 165–167
nontraditional, 11–12,
 81–82, 231–232
physical comfort in, 85,
 98–100

predictability in, 80, 82,
 84–90, 96–98
respectful dialogue in,
 35–36, 85, 102–104,
 154–156
self-disclosure in, 84,
 90–93, 201
time boundaries in, 84,
 86–88
Clinical courses, 10, 171–202
abnormal behavior,
 180–183
clinical seminars, 11–12,
 125–132, 193–202
projective testing, 173–180
psychoanalytic theory and
 therapy, 183–193
Clinical field training, 10,
 192–193, 200–202
Clinical material used in
 classes, 90–92, 193–197,
 244–249, 261–271
Clinical seminars, 11–12,
 125–132, 193–202
Clinical supervision
in academic institutions,
 11–12
ambiguity accommodated
 in, 41–42
competes with teaching,
 200–202
literature on, 11–12
psychoanalytic paradigm
 in, 192–193
Cohler, B. J., 22
Competency concerns,
 20–21, 221–224
Competition among students,
 260–261

Complementary
    identification, 37–38,
    161–162
Concordant identification,
    37, 161–162
Confidentiality
    in classroom, 82, 85–86,
        106–108, 157
    in therapeutic frame, 80
Containment, 39–40,
    239–240
Countertransference. *See also*
    Transference
    benign, 198–199
    in classroom, 148–160,
        197–200, 240–242
    hostile, 199–200
    neutrality and, 150–151
    overprotective, 197–198
    projective identification
        and, 160–167
    rejecting, 199
    selective attention, 241
    talking down, 240–241
    teaching about, 188
    in therapy, 148–150
Course evaluations, 86,
    108–110, 275–276
Course preparation. *See*
    Preparation
Course syllabi, 84, 89–90,
    144
Criticality, 214
Curiosity, 33–34

Davis, B. G., 89–90
Deadlines, 144–155
Dependence on authority,
    20–21, 127, 259–260

Depression, childhood, 25
Depressive character style,
    219–220
Diagnosis. *See also* Projective
    testing
    of learning problems,
        25–26
    of psychiatric conditions,
        180–183
Disclosure, 244–245. *See also*
    Confidentiality;
    Self-disclosure
Disturbing imagery, 182–183
Drive theory. *See*
    Psychosexuality

Ebel, K. E., 78, 231
Eber, M., 31
Edwards, R., 8–9
Ego functions, 20, 119–120,
    127–128
Ego psychology, 119–120,
    127–128, 174
Ekstein, R., 13–16
Empathy
    development of, 36–38,
        121–124
    learning disability and,
        25–26
    in lecturing, 236–237
    and motive to learn, 21–23
    and motive to teach and
        help, 36–38
    in psychoanalytic therapy,
        36–38, 187–188
    in self psychology, 21–23,
        121–124
Ethical issues, 39–40, 49–50,
    100–102, 155–160, 202

Evaluation, 253–276. *See also*
    Diagnosis; Projective
    testing
    assumptions underlying,
        257–261
    as clinical process,
        261–271
    compared to projective
        testing, 257
    examples of tests, 263–271
    feedback from, 275–276
    grading, 271–275
    interpersonal dynamics
        during, 96–98,
        254–261
    test formats, 261–263
Extensions on assignments,
    36, 144–145
Extrainstructional contacts
    in classroom frame, 85,
        100–102
    student-initiated, 145–146
    teacher-initiated, 156–157

Family background
    of practitioners, 31–32,
        36–38, 40–42, 182
    of students, 19–21, 24–25
Favoritism, 198–199, 241
Feedback
    student, 42, 108–110,
        275–276
    teacher, 84–85, 93–98,
        271–275
Fees, 80, 82, 85, 104–106
Field, K., 7–9
Field training, 200–202
    analytic model in, 10,
        192–193

Figure-drawing tests, 173
Framework. *See* Classroom
    frame; Therapeutic frame
Freud, Anna
    on childhood education, 14
    on teaching and
        psychoanalysis, 5, 77
Freud, Sigmund
    on psychoanalysis, 78
    on psychosexuality,
        115–116
    on self-disclosure, 90
    on teaching, 5
    terminology of, 116–117
    on therapeutic frame,
        79–81
    on transference, 138–139

Garber, B., 25–26
Gill, M. M., 138–139, 142
Glickauf-Hughes, C., 123–124
Goldberg, C., 31
Good-enough mothering,
    56–58
Good-enough schools, 58–71
Grade modification,
    158–160, 274–275
Graded work
    self-disclosure in, 92–93
    teacher feedback on, 93–98
    timely return of, 96–98
Grades
    competition for, 260–261
    conflict around, 154–156,
        272–273
Grading
    criteria, 154–156, 271–275
    ethical issues in, 155–156

Grading (*continued*)
  psychoanalytic perspective
    on, 273–275
  test format and, 271–272
Grandiose self, 238–239, 260
Greer, J. M., 25
Ground rules. *See* Classroom
    frame; Therapeutic frame
Guy, J. D., 31–32

Hartmann, H., 119–120
Historical background, 5–6,
    12–17
Holding environment. *See
    also* Classroom frame
  academic institution as,
    58–71
  as psychoanalytic
    construct, 55–58
Hostile countertransference,
    199–200
Hysterical character style,
    218–219

Idea pool, 8–9
Idealization, 16, 121,
    123–124
  of teachers, 16, 21–22,
    175–176
Identification, 194–197,
    215–216, 274
  with clients, 37–38,
    178–180, 184
  projective, 160–167
Inappropriate behavior
  by students, 145, 162–164
  by teachers, 102–104,
    154–156, 199–200,
    240–242

Indirect communication,
    146–147, 157
Infant development, 56–58,
    115–116
Inhibition, 122
Interpersonal processes. *See
  also* Intrapsychic
  processes
  countertransference
    benign, 198–199
    in classroom, 148–160,
      197–200, 240–242
    construct, 148–150
    hostile, 199–200
    neutrality and, 150–151
    overprotective, 197–198
    projective identification
      and, 160–167
    rejecting, 199
    selective attention, 241
    talking down, 240–241
    teaching about, 188
    in therapy, 148–150
  intrapsychic processes and,
    135–138
  projective identification
    in classroom, 161–167
    construct, 160–161
  transference
    in classroom, 16, 20,
      140–148, 160–167
    construct, 138–140
    identification of, 142–147
    interventions, 147–148
    neutrality and, 139–142
    projective identification
      and, 160–167
    in therapy, 39–40, 45–46
    types of, 142–143

Intimacy, 43–45, 49–50
Intrapsychic processes,
    113–132
  ego functions, 20,
    119–120, 127–128
  interpersonal processes
    and, 135–138
  object relations, 19–21,
    120–121, 128–129
  psychosexuality, 115–119
  classroom dynamics and,
    18–19, 117–119,
    127, 131–132
  construct, 115–116
  learning and, 18–19,
    23–24, 116–119,
    127, 131–132
  in motivation to teach
    and help, 31
  selfobject needs, 21–23,
    121–124, 129–131

Jones, Richard, 5

Kaley, H., 7
Kaye, S., 25
Kernberg, O., 60–61
Klein, Emanuel, 24
Kolstoe, O. P., 42
Kris, Ernst, 12–13, 15
Kunz, L. B., 31

Langs, R., 78–79, 81–82,
    139–140, 158
Language, 116, 188–190
Leadership, 60–61
Learning
  countertransference
    impedes, 150–167,
    197–200, 240–242

  ego functions and, 20, 120,
    127–128
  motivation of, 17–23
  object relations and,
    19–21, 121, 128–129
  psychosexuality and,
    18–19, 23–24,
    116–119, 127,
    131–132
  self-object needs and,
    21–23, 122–124,
    129–130
Learning alliance, 16
Learning problems
  neurological basis of,
    24–26
  psychological basis of,
    20–21, 23–26, 122,
    143–148, 179–180
Lecturing, 231–249
  content of, 242–249
  contrasted to
    psychoanalytic
    therapy, 232–236
  countertransference in,
    240–242
  directive nature of,
    233–235
  disclosure in, 244–245
  empathetic, 236–237
  interpersonal dynamics in,
    242–244
  psychological vulnerability
    in, 237–240
  value of, 231–232
Lerner, P., 114
Liss, Edward, 24
Listening skills, 33–37,
    102–103

Literature on psychoanalysis
    and education, 5–26
  on classroom teaching,
    8–12
  general, 5–7
  new developments in, 6–9,
    77–78
  teacher's role developed in,
    12–17, 77–78
Lunardi, P. M., 81

Managed care, 191–192
Maroda, K., 140
Math disability, 25
Mehlman, E., 123–124
Mentoring relationship. See
    Classroom dynamics
Mirroring, 121, 123–124
Misperceptions about
    psychoanalysis, 184–188
Mothers, 56–58
Motive to learn, 17–23
Motive to teach and help
  components of, 32–45
  origins in family
    background, 31–32,
    36–38, 40–42, 182
  psychological risks
    associated with, 46–51
Motto, R. L., 13–16

Narcissistic character style,
    220–221
Neurological impairment,
    25–26
Neutrality
  analytic, 39–40, 90,
    139–140, 149–150

teacher, 140–142,
    150–151, 239–240
Nonverbal behaviors,
    162–164

Oberdornf, C. P., 23
Object relations, 120–121,
    128–129
  in learning development
    models, 19–21
  projective identification
    and, 160–165
  projective testing and, 174
Obsessive-compulsive
    character style, 217–218
Organizational dynamics,
    58–66, 104–106,
    165–166
Outpatient clinics, 192–193
Overanalysis, 185–187
Overprotective
    countertransference,
    197–198

Parent–child relationship,
    19–23, 56–58, 121–124
Peller, Lili, 19
Personality dynamics. See
    Intrapsychic processes
Personality theory, 217–221
Physical comfort, 85, 98–100
Physical security, 66–67
Pine, F., 114–115
Postmodernism, 8–9
Power, 45–46, 118–119,
    256–260
Predictability
  in academic institutions,
    65–66

in classroom frame, 80, 82,
    84–90, 96–98
in therapeutic frame, 79–81
Preparation, 207–228
    administrators influence,
        224–228
    character styles and,
        216–221
    as clinical process,
        207–210
    competency concerns and,
        221–224
    criticality and, 214
    lack of, 153–154
    psychological vulnerability
        in, 212–214
    regression in, 211–214
    role models influence,
        215–216
    students influence,
        221–224, 226
Professional identity
    in academic institutions, 29
    ambiguity and, 40–42
    challenges to forming
        integrated, 29,
        272–276
    curiosity and, 33–34
    empathy and, 36–38
    family background
        influences, 31–32,
        36–38, 40–42
    intimacy and, 43–45
    listening skills and, 33–37
    motivation and, 30–46
    power and, 45–46
    psychological hardship and,
        31–32, 36–38, 40–42,
        182

psychological risks to,
    46–51
role models and, 215–216
self-denial and, 38–40
Projective identification. See
    also
    Countertransference;
    Transference
    in classroom, 161–167
    construct, 160–161
Projective testing, 173–174
    compared to classroom
        testing, 257
    teaching, 174–180
Psychoanalytic constructs,
    113–116, 119–124,
    138–140, 148–150,
    161–162. See also
    Interpersonal processes;
    Intrapsychic processes
Psychoanalytic framework.
    See Classroom frame;
    Therapeutic frame
Psychoanalytic supervision.
    See Clinical supervision
Psychoanalytic theory and
    therapy courses,
    183–193
Psychoanalytic therapy,
    209–210
    ambiguity in, 40–42
    contrasted to teaching,
        40–42, 232–236
    dangers to therapists in,
        47–50
    empathy in, 36–38,
        187–188
    frame in, 78–81
    intimacy in, 43

Psychoanalytic therapy
  (*continued*)
  intrapsychic processes in,
    113–115
  listening in, 33–35
  misperceptions of,
    184–188
  responses to clients in,
    38–40
  transference in, 39–40,
    45–46
Psychosexuality
  classroom dynamics and,
    18–19, 117–119, 127,
    131–132
  construct, 115–116
  learning and, 18–19,
    23–24, 116–119, 127,
    131–132
  in motivation to teach and
    help, 31
Publication material, 61–62

Questions from students,
  242–244

Reactions to clients, model
  of, 38
Reading disability, 25
Reality testing, 120–122
Regression, 211–214
Rejecting
  countertransference, 199
Respectful dialogue, 33–37,
  85, 102–104, 154–156
Responses to psychoanalytic
  therapy clients, 39–40
Role models, 67–68
  shortage of, 10–11

for teachers, 10–11, 67,
  215–216
teachers as, 44–45, 67–68,
  90–91
Role play, 81
Rorschach test, 173, 175–177

Safe learning environment,
  62–63, 108–110,
  194–197, 224–225
Salaries, 85, 104–106
Salzberger-Wittenberg, I., 44
Scapegoating, 241
Schafer, R., 257
School problems. *See*
  Inappropriate behavior;
  Learning problems
Schools. *See* Academic
  institutions; Classroom
  frame
Selective attention, 241
Self psychology, 21–23,
  121–124, 128–129
  projective testing and, 174
Self representations, 120–121
Self-absorption, 51–52
Self-denial, 38–40
Self-diagnosis, 181–182
Self-disclosure, 84, 90–93,
  201
  by teachers, 90–92,
    126–127, 131–132,
    244–249
Self-esteem, 22, 123
Selfobject needs, 21–23,
  121–124, 129–130
Selfobjects, 21
Self-processing, 81

Seminars. *See* Clinical seminars
Sexual abuse, 25, 100
Sexual harassment, 100
Shore, K., 191
Shulman, M. E., 191
Shur, R., 9, 60–61, 165
Silence, 34–35, 39
Smith, D. L., 78, 90, 100, 139–140
Social contacts. *See* Extrainstructional contacts
Stupidity, 23
Sublimation, 19
Submission to authority, 258–259
Supervision. *See* Clinical supervision
Sutherland, R. L., 117–119, 127
Syllabi, 84, 89–90, 144

Talking down to students, 240–241
Tansey, M. J., 38, 161–162
Tardiness
 by students, 143–145
 by teachers, 86–88, 97–98, 152–153
Teacher intervention, 130–132, 147–148, 158–160, 165–167, 236–237
Teacher neutrality, 140–142, 150–151, 239–240
Teaching tasks. *See* Evaluation; Lecturing; Preparation

Terminology, 116–117, 188–190
Test anxiety, 255–261
Test format, 261–271
 examples of, 263–271
Testing. *See* Evaluation; Projective testing
Thematic apperception test (TAT), 173
Theoretical orientation, 10, 192–193
Therapeutic frame, 78–81, 100, 158. *See also* Classroom frame
 in clinic setting, 192–193
Therapy. *See* Psychoanalytic therapy
Thompson, R., 10
Time boundaries, 80, 82, 84, 86–88
Time management, 96–98, 143–145, 152–153
Transference. *See also* Countertransference
 in classroom, 16, 20, 140–148, 160–167
 construct, 138–140
 identification of, 142–147
 interventions, 147–148
 neutrality and, 139–142
 projective identification and, 160–167
 in therapy, 39–40, 45–46
 types of, 142–143
Treatment setting. *See* Therapeutic frame
Troise, F. P., 140
Tuition, 104
Twinship needs, 121, 123–124

Usher, R., 8–9

Victimization, 161–167, 179
Vlosky, M., 193
Voyeuristic conflict, 25

Winnicott, D. W., 56–58
Wisdom figures, 174–176
Wisocki, P. A., 10, 47
Wolf, E. S., 22–23
Wool, G. F., 16

ABOUT THE AUTHOR

Jed A. Yalof, Psy. D., is Chair of the Graduate Psychology Department, Immaculata College, Immaculata, Pennsylvania, where he is also a professor and Director of Counseling and Testing Services. He maintains a private practice in clinical and school psychology in Narberth, Pennsylvania.